Trauma and Emergency Surgery

Edited by Selim Sözen
and Burhan Hakan Kanat

Published in London, United Kingdom

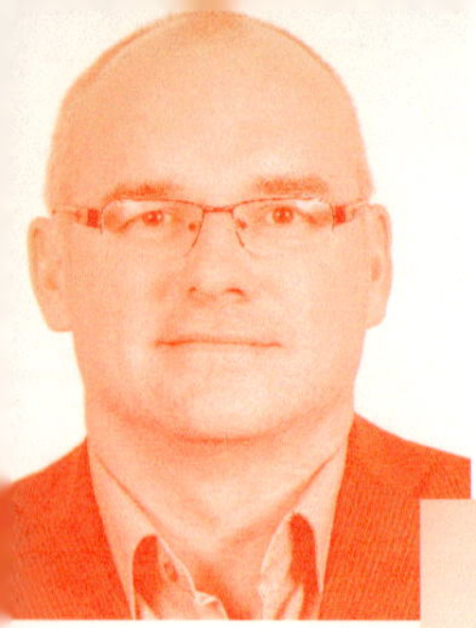

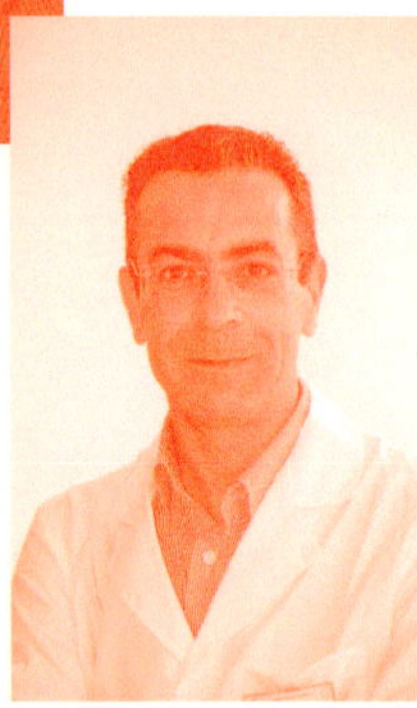

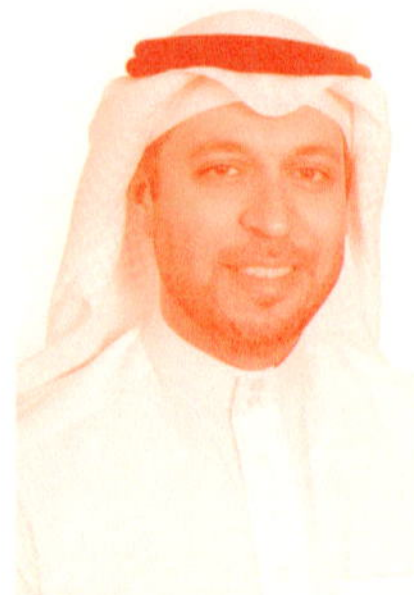

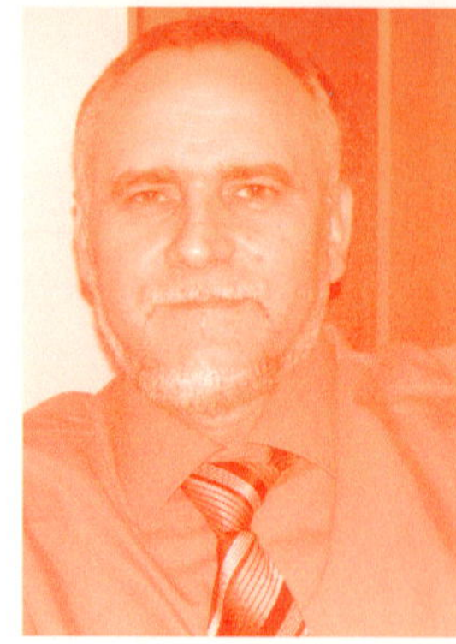

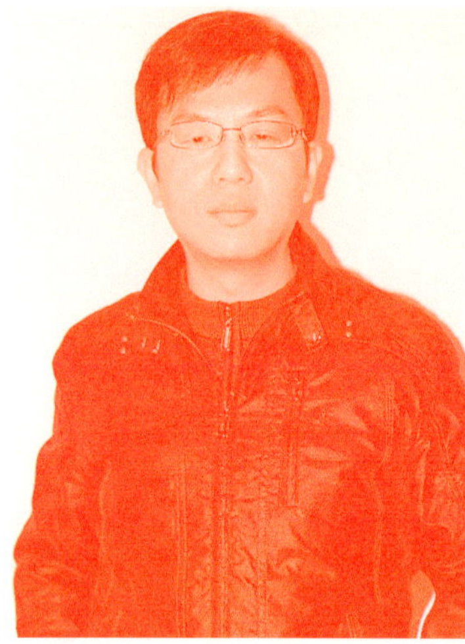

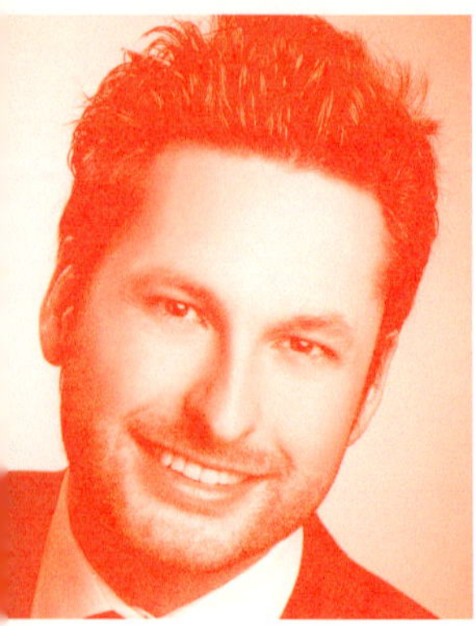

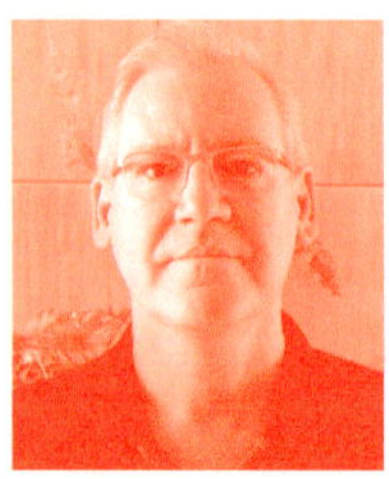

IntechOpen

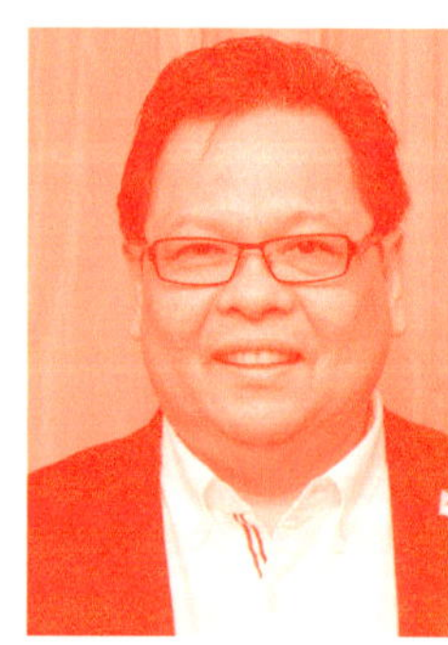

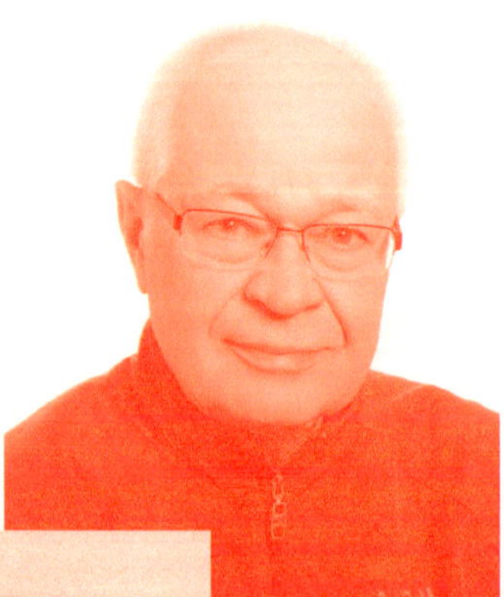

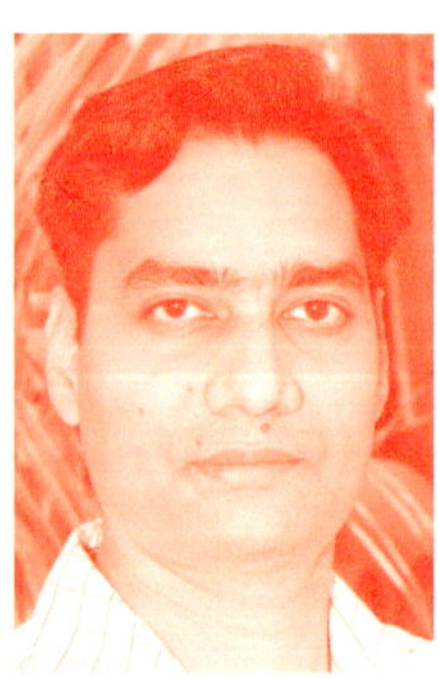

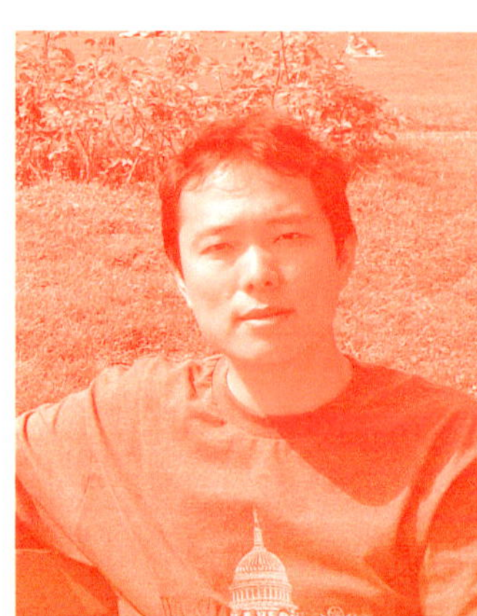

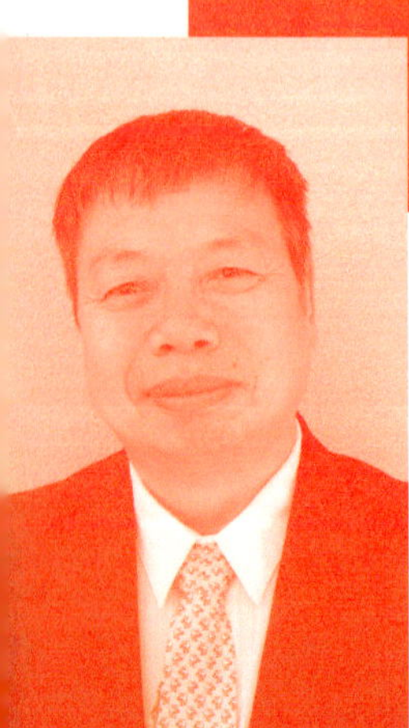

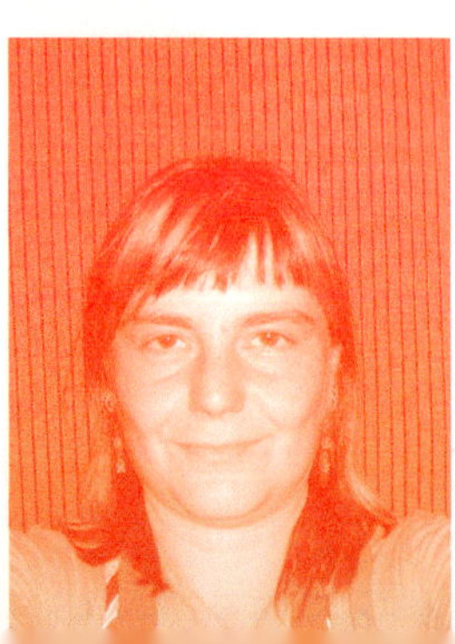

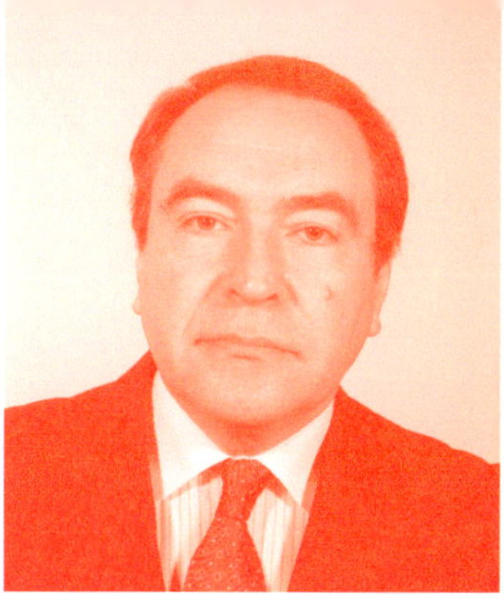
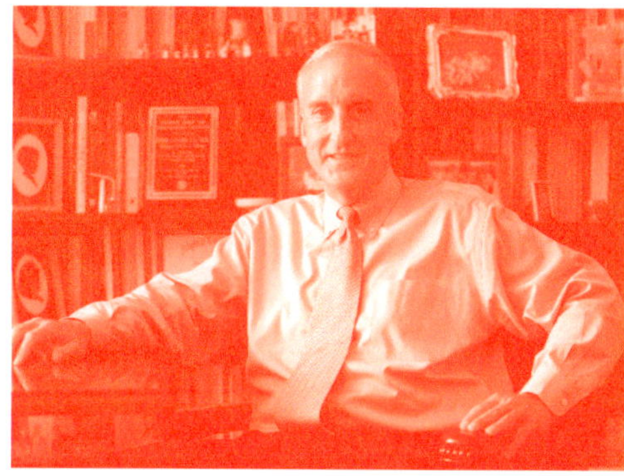
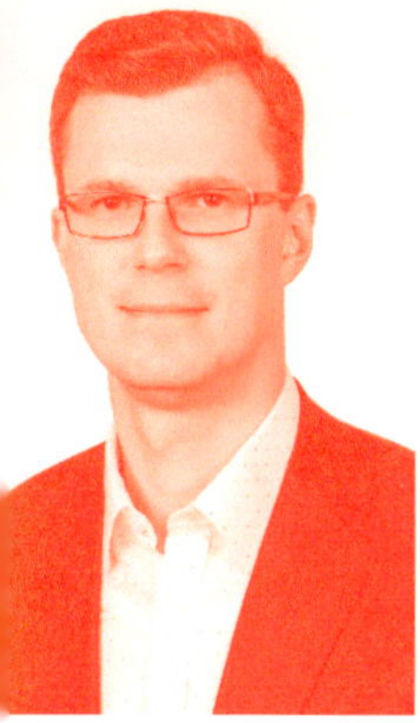
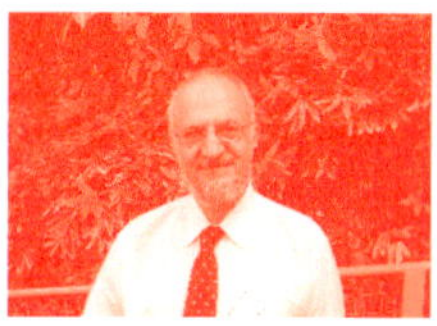
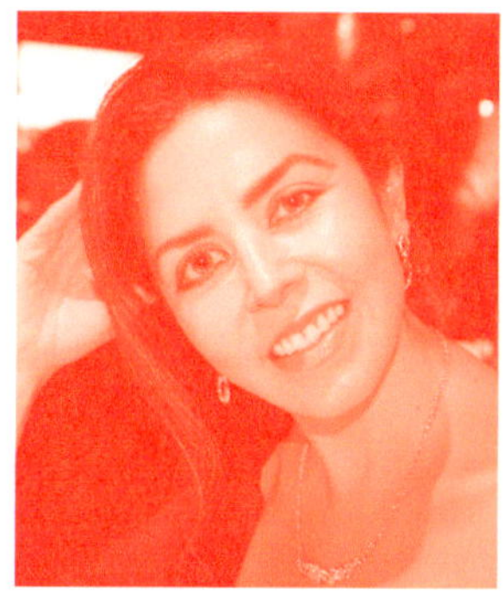

Supporting open minds since 2005

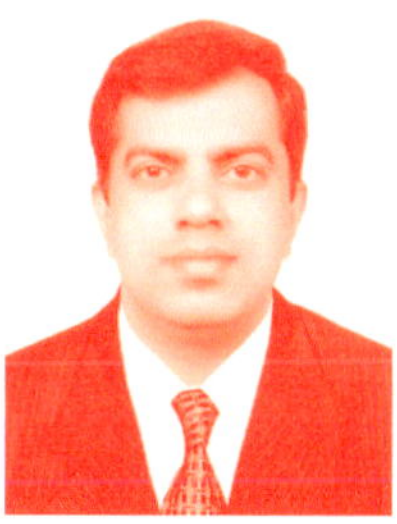
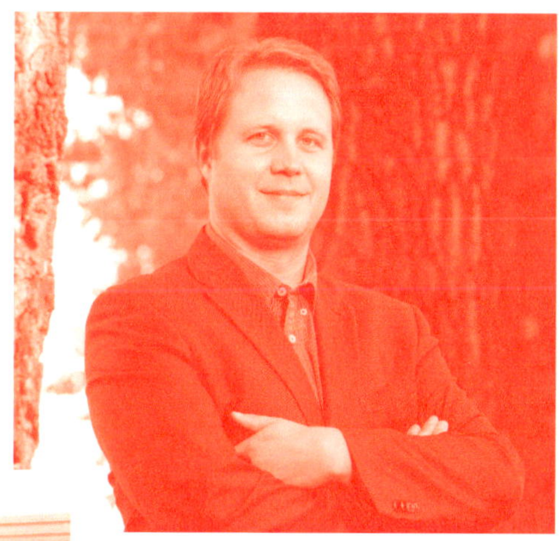
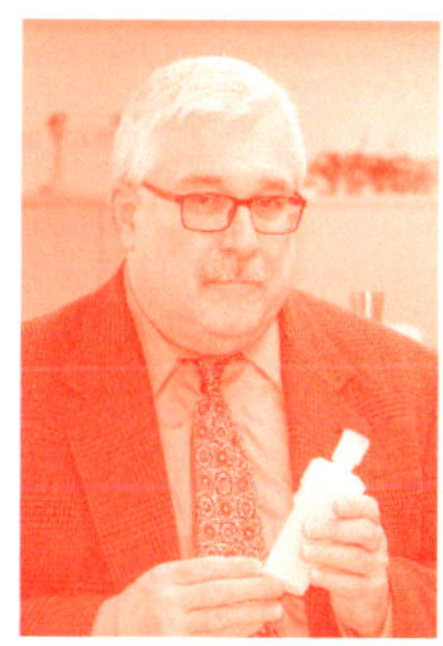
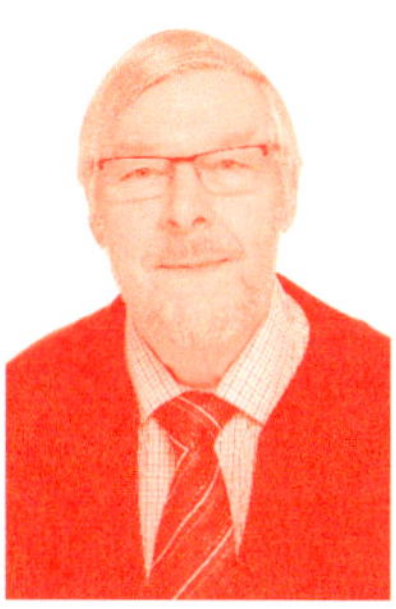
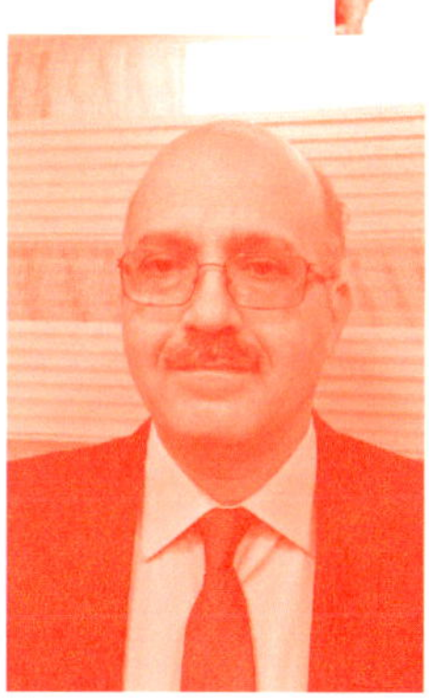
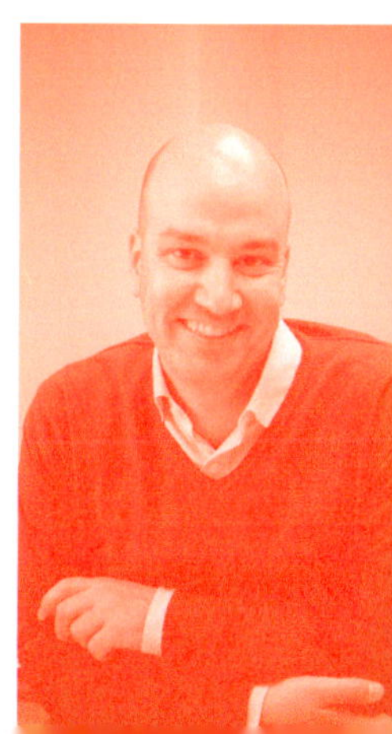
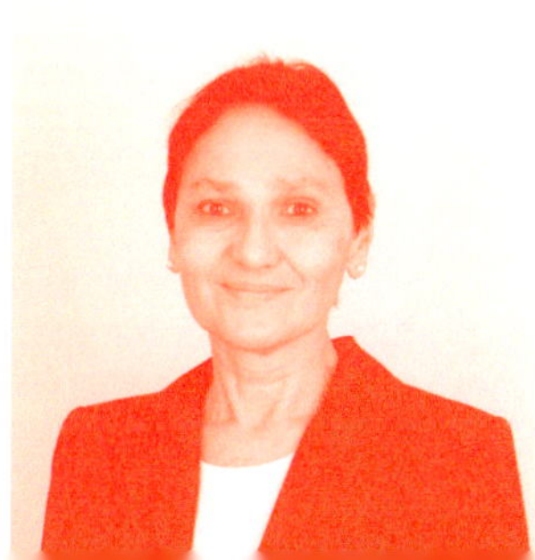

Trauma and Emergency Surgery
http://dx.doi.org/10.5772/intechopen.94683
Edited by Selim Sözen and Burhan Hakan Kanat

Contributors
Alex Pontini, Bruno Azzena, Filippo Andrea Giovanni Perozzo, Alvise Montanari, Alberto De Lazzari, Giovanni Valotto, Tuba Apaydın, Pabitha Devi B. Mehanathan, Subash Mehta, Athisayamani Giftson, Reesha Pa, Turkan Dubus, Soe Wunna Htay, Balaji Zacharia, Raj Vignesh, Domenico Calcaterra, Selim Sözen, Serhat Doğan, Burhan Hakan Kanat, Gökhan Söğütlü, Mehmet Gencturk, Hasan Erdem

First published in London, United Kingdom, 2022 by IntechOpen
IntechOpen is the global imprint of INTECHOPEN LIMITED, registered in England and Wales, registration number: 11086078, 5 Princes Gate Court, London, SW7 2QJ, United Kingdom
Printed in Croatia

British Library Cataloguing-in-Publication Data
A catalogue record for this book is available from the British Library

Additional hard and PDF copies can be obtained from orders@intechopen.com

Trauma and Emergency Surgery
Edited by Selim Sözen and Burhan Hakan Kanat
p. cm.
Print ISBN 978-1-83969-523-0
Online ISBN 978-1-83969-524-7
eBook (PDF) ISBN 978-1-83969-525-4

For EU product safety concerns:
IN TECH d.o.o., Prolaz Marije Krucifikse Kozulić 3, 51000 Rijeka, Croatia, info@intechopen.com or visit our website at intechopen.com.

Meet the editors

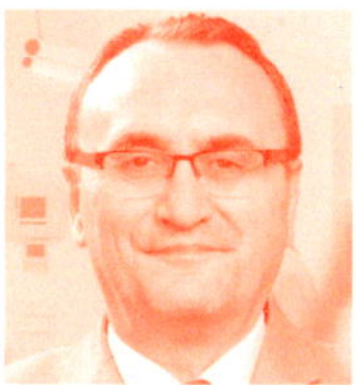

Dr. Selim Sözen is an expert in general surgery who received his medical degree from Ondokuz Mayıs University, Turkey, in 1998. From 1999 to 2004, he was an assistant doctor at Ankara Atatürk Education and Research Hospital, Turkey. From 2004 to 2013, he worked as a specialist at different government hospitals in Turkey. He joined the Department of General Surgery, Medicine Faculty, Namık Kemal University, Turkey, as an associate professor in 2013. He completed liver transplantation surgery at İnönü University, Turkey, in 2014–2015. Since 2016, Dr. Sözen has run his own surgery clinic in İstanbul, Turkey. He is a member of the Turkish Surgical Association and a review board member for several journals. He has published 105 articles in scientific journals and presented 64 poster papers at scientific congresses. His research interests include general, gastrointestinal, emergency, and trauma surgery, bacterial translocation, liver disease, and hernia surgery.

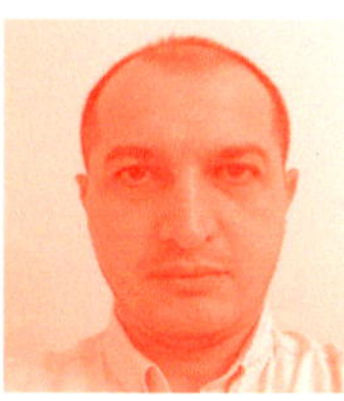

Dr. Burhan Hakan Kanat graduated from the Faculty of Medicine, İnönü University, Turkey, in 2005. He trained in general surgery at the Faculty of Medicine, Fırat University, Turkey, in 2011. He also worked as a specialist at the Elazığ Training and Research Hospital, Turkey. In 2013, he received a Certificate of Surgical Competence from the Turkish Surgery Society. He completed liver transplantation surgery at İnönü University in 2014–2015. He received training in breast-endocrine surgery in 2016. Dr. Kanat joined the Department of General Surgery, Medicine Faculty, Health Sciences University, Turkey, as an associate professor in 2017–2020. Since October 2020, he has been an associate professor at the Department of General Surgery, Medicine Faculty, Malatya Turgut Özal University, Turkey. He is a member of the Turkish Surgical Society, International Pilonidal Society, and Turkish Society of Colon and Rectal Surgery. Since October 2020, he has been an associate professor at the Department of General Surgery, Medicine Faculty, Malatya Turgut Özal University, Turkey. Dr. Kanat is an author of more than 100 publications including five book chapters. He is also a review board member for several journals.

Contents

Preface

This book is a collection of review papers on trauma and emergency surgery. In addition to sharing their knowledge, the authors provide their personal clinical experience, making this book a useful resource for scientists and physicians practicing in the field of trauma and emergency surgery. The book is divided into six sections with chapters showing the application of different surgical specialties.

In Section 1, Chapter 1, "Blunt Abdominal Injury", Dr. B. Mehanathan Pabithandevi et al. discusses blunt abdominal injuries. In Chapter 2, "Rectus Sheath Hematoma", Dr. Selim Sözen et al. discuss the types and treatment of rectus sheath hematoma, an uncommon and often clinically misdiagnosed cause of abdominal pain. In the second section, Chapter 3, "Blunt Traumatic Aortic Injury" Domenico Calcaterra examines thoracic endovascular aortic replacement (TEVAR) as the new standard for treating TAIs. TEVAR is associated with a lower risk of operative mortality; however, the optimal timing for delivering this therapy remains unclear with respect to identifying patients who require immediate intervention versus those for whom postponing treatment of the aortic injury would be preferable.

In Section 3, Chapter 4, "The Role of Minimally Invasive Surgery in Management of Chest Trauma," Dr. Apaydın Tuba focuses on chest trauma and the use of video thoracoscopy as a safe and beneficial diagnostic and therapeutic device in select patients with chest trauma with no indication for emergent thoracotomy or sternotomy. Video thoracoscopy is also beneficial in the acute or retarded approach for patients with blunt chest trauma for treatment of clotted hemothorax, persistent pneumothorax, thoracic empyema, and chylothorax, as well as for diagnosis of diaphragmatic injuries. Chapter 5, "Surgical Approach to Rib Fractures" by Dr. Dubus Turkan, examines rib fractures and their surgical stabilization, which reduces possible pulmonary complications in patients. Surgery shortens the duration of hospital stay and the time to return to work as well as improves patient quality of life by physiologically improving breathing.

In Section 4, Chapter 6, "Management of Traumatic Brain Injury," Soe Wunna Htay provides information about the approach to traumatic brain injuries. Section 5, includes Chapter 7, "Acute Compartment Syndrome of the Extremities and Paraspinal Muscles" by Dr. Zacharia Balaji and Raj Vignesh Selvaraj which discusses the etiologies, clinical features, investigations, and management of acute compartment syndrome of the extremities and the paraspinal region.

In Section 6, Chapter 8, "Management and Clinical Aspects of Burned Patients Affected by SARS-COV2," Dr. Alex Pontini et al., discusses COVID-19 infection in burn patients.

I thank the authors for their professional dedication and outstanding work in summarizing their clinical and research practices.

Selim Sözen
Associate Professor of General Surgery,
Sözen Surgery Clinic,
İstanbul, Turkey

Burhan Hakan Kanat
Malatya Turgut Özal University,
Turkey

Section 1

Abdominal Surgery and Trauma

Chapter 1

Blunt Abdominal Injury

Pabithadevi B. Mehanathan, Subash Metha, Athisayamani Jeyapaul and Reesha Pa

Abstract

Road traffic accidents are one of the leading causes of mortality. Blunt injury to the abdomen contributes to mortality second to head injury. The mechanism of injury in road traffic accidents is due to blunt force created by collision between the patient and the external forces and acceleration and deceleration forces acting on the person's internal forces. The common solid organs involved in blunt abdominal trauma are the spleen, liver, and kidney. Mesenteric tears and isolated small bowel injuries can also occur. A high degree of suspicion and watchfulness, regular examination, imaging, and investigations are needed to diagnose blunt abdominal injury. The eFAST exam is an emergency screening tool used to diagnose intra-abdominal injuries in emergency departments. Treatment for these injuries depends on hemodynamic status, whether stable or unstable. Hemodynamically unstable patients with a positive eFAST exam will be taken up for emergency exploration, while stable patients will undergo further imaging and investigation to plan management. This chapter discusses the grades of injuries in the spleen, liver, mesentery, and retroperitoneum. It also discusses the various diagnostic and treatment modalities available and when and where to use them. This chapter is useful for surgical postgraduates, aspiring surgeons, and trauma surgeons.

Keywords: blunt abdominal injury, AAST grading, splenic injury, liver injury, retroperitoneal hematoma

1. Introduction

Abdominal blunt injury is a common emergency in emergency departments that regularly results from road traffic accidents, assaults, or accidental falls. Since the occurrence of road traffic accidents is increasing, they are now the leading cause of global disease burdens. According to the 2013 Global Status Report on Road Safety, more than 1.3 lakh people died on Indian roads, giving India the dubious honour of topping the global risk of fatalities from road crashes. Head injury, fractures, and blunt abdominal injury are the common causes of death in road traffic accident injuries.

2. Mechanism of blunt abdominal injury

Intra-abdominal injuries secondary to blunt force are due to collisions between the injured person and external forces and the acceleration and deceleration forces acting on the person's internal organs.

2.1 Deceleration

Rapid deceleration causes differentiating movement among adjacent structures. As a result, shear forces are created and cause injury to hollow, solid visceral organs and vascular pedicles at relatively fixed points of attachment, for example, a hepatic tear along the ligamentum teres. As bowel loops travel from their mesenteric attachments, mesenteric tears with resultant splanchnic vessel injuries can result.

2.2 Crushing

Intra-abdominal contents can be crushed between the anterior abdominal and vertebral columns. Solid viscera such as the spleen, liver, and kidneys are more vulnerable to crush injuries.

2.3 External compression

External compressive forces such as direct blows or external compression against a fixed object result in a sudden and dramatic rise in intra-abdominal pressure, which can cause a rupture of the hollow viscus, in accordance with the principles of Boyle's law. The liver, spleen, small intestine, and large intestine are the most frequently injured organs in increasing order of frequency.

3. Clinical examination

Abdominal blunt injury is associated with other injuries, such as head injuries or fractures, thus the presenting symptom will vary. For blunt injury alone, the patient will present with abdominal distension, abdominal pain, or hemodynamic instability.

Once the patient enters the emergency room, a primary survey is performed. Primary survey consists of:

- Airway
- Breathing—oxygen saturation
- Circulation—pulse rate, volume, and blood pressure
- Glasgow coma scale

Abdominal examination follows the primary survey and includes:

- Inspection—pattern contusions, abrasion, abdominal distension
- Palpation—tenderness, guarding, rigidity, rib fracture, pelvic fracture
- Percussion—for free fluid and liver dullness obliteration
- Auscultation—bowel sounds

After primary examinations, clear the airway, resuscitate for breathing (if necessary), and insert a wide-bore IV needle for infusion or insert a central venous catheter. According to the Advanced Trauma Life Support (ATLS) definition, a patient is "unstable" with blood pressure < 90 mmHg and heart rate > 120 bpm, evidence of skin vasoconstriction (cool, clammy, decreased capillary refill), altered level of consciousness, and/or shortness of breath.

If the patient is hemodynamically unstable, stabilize first with crystalloids, colloids, or blood transfusion (whichever is applicable) and perform an eFAST exam. If there is any evidence of free fluid, the patient is shifted directly to emergency operation theatre (EOT). If the patient is hemodynamically stable and the primary survey is negative, the patient can be shifted to CT scan and review. A strong suspicion is needed to diagnose blunt injury in the abdomen.

4. Splenic injury

Splenic injury is the most common visceral injury from violence. The likelihood of severe injury is increased in a diseased spleen.

Splenic injury is commonly associated with the left hemothorax, fracture of the left lower ribs, and injuries to the tail of the pancreas, left lobe of the liver, left kidney, or left colon. Direct compression of the spleen causes parenchymal injury. Rapid deceleration causes tears to splenic parenchyma. Direct blows to the abdomen (domestic violence or leisure and play activities) can also cause splenic rupture.

4.1 Clinical presentation

- Hilar injury: rapid development of shock and rapid deterioration (even death can occur).

- Other injuries: features of shock (pallor, tachycardia, restlessness, tachypnea, anxiety, hypotension, decreased capillary refill, and decreased pulse pressure).

- Abdominal pain, distension, tenderness, and abdominal rigidity in the left upper quadrant (LUQ); positive Kehr's sign (a clot or blood collected under the left diaphragm that irritates it and the phrenic nerve (C3, C4) causing referred pain in left shoulder 15 min after foot end elevation).

- Delayed splenic rupture (DSR): latent period of Baudet in which the patient has no signs or symptoms for hours to days and presents later. DSR tends to occur 4–8 days after trauma. This may be due to expanding subcapsular hematoma, clot disruption, pseudocyst rupture, or pseudoaneurysm/AV fistula rupture (**Table 1**).

4.2 Management of splenic injury

Management of splenic injury depends on the hemodynamic stability of the patient and associated injuries. It can be managed nonoperatively, operatively, or via splenic artery angioembolization.

Patients who have diffuse peritonitis or who are hemodynamically unstable (a positive FAST examination or positive diagnostic peritoneal lavage (DPL)) following blunt abdominal trauma should be taken urgently for exploratory laparotomy. A routine laparotomy is not indicated in hemodynamically stable patients without peritonitis presenting with isolated splenic injury. Factors such as patient age, grade of injury, and presence of hypotension need to be considered in the clinical management of these patients. For patients undergoing nonoperative management (NOM), an abdominal CT scan with IV contrast should be performed to identify and assess the severity of injury to the spleen. Angiography should be considered for patients with AAST grade

Grade	Type of injury	Description
I	Laceration Hematoma	Capsular tear, <1 cm depth Involving <10% TSA of spleen
II	Laceration Hematoma	1–3 cm parenchymal depth which does not involve a trabecular vessel Subcapsular, Involving 10–50% TSA of spleen, Intra parenchymal, <5 cm in depth
III	Laceration Hematoma	>3 cm parencymal depth or involving trabecular vessels Subcapsular involving >50% of TSA of spleen or expanding; ruptured subcapsular or parenchymal hematoma
IV	Laceration	Segmental or hilar (>25% devascularization)
V	Laceration Vascular	Shattered spleen Hilar vascular injury which devascularizes the spleen

Table 1.
American Association for the Surgery of Trauma (AAST) splenic injury scale.

III injuries. The presence of a contrast blush, moderate hemoperitoneum, or evidence of ongoing splenic bleeding is an indication for splenectomy. Nonoperative management of splenic injuries should only be considered in an environment that provides capabilities for continuous monitoring, such as serial clinical evaluations, serial HB estimation, serial radiological screening, and availability of an emergency operating room at any given time [1]. If vital signs or hematocrit values decrease, or if there is evidence of expanding hematoma or ongoing bleeding, the patient should be shifted for emergency laparotomy.

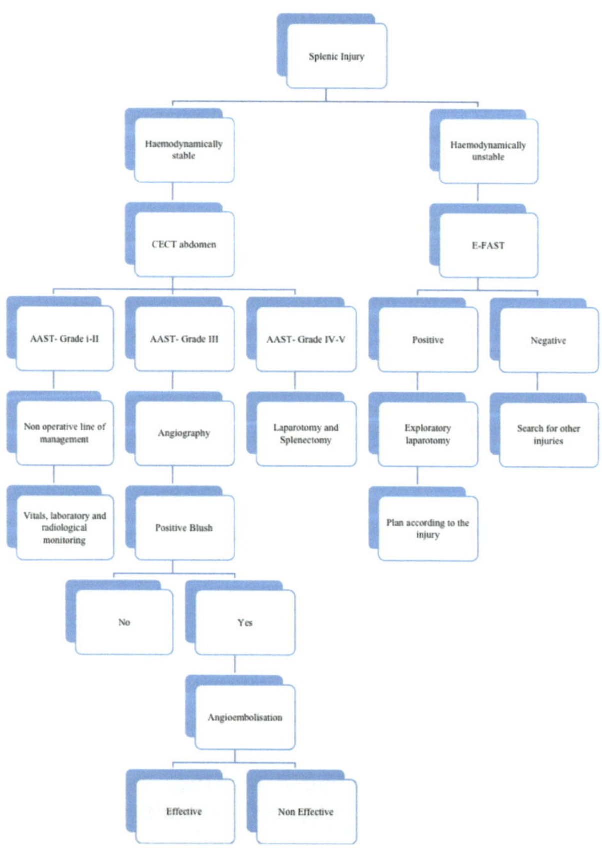

5. Liver injury

The liver is the most common organ injured in blunt and penetrating injuries. Its anterior location in the abdomen and fragile parenchyma makes it susceptible to injury from blunt forces. Its fixed location under the diaphragm also makes it susceptible to shear forces from deceleration injuries. The vasculature in the liver is made up of large but thin-walled vessels with high blood flow (**Table 2**).

5.1 Nonoperative management (NOM) of traumatic liver injury

Blunt trauma patients with hemodynamic stability and absence of other internal injuries requiring surgery can be treated nonoperatively. Patients can undergo NOM irrespective of the grade of liver injury. NOM should not be used for patients with hemodynamic instability and peritonitis. NOM should be adopted in centers with facilities for intensive care monitoring, angiography, immediate availability of an operating room, and immediate access to blood products [2, 3]. CT angiogram should be performed in patients considered for NOM. If there is any blush in the CT angiogram, angioembolization should be considered. NOM patients should be continuously monitored for vitals, hematocrit, abdominal girth, and the development of peritonitis.

Complications of NOM include:

- bleeding
- abdominal compartment syndrome
- infections (abscesses and other infections)
- biliary complications (bile leak, hemobilia, bilioma, biliary peritonitis, biliary fistula) [2, 3]
- liver necrosis
- rebleeding or secondary hemorrhage (rupture of a subcapsular hematoma or a pseudoaneurysm)

Grade	Type of injury	Description
I	Laceration Hematoma	<1 cm depth, nonbleeding Subcapsular, Nonexpanding, Involving <10% TSA of liver
II	Laceration Hematoma	1–3 cm depth, <10 cm in length Subcapsular, Involving 10–50% TSA, nonexpanding
III	Laceration Hematoma	>3 cm depth Subcapsular—involving >50% of TSA, intraparenchymal >2 cm, expanding
IV	Hematoma Laceration	Bleeding intraparenchymal rupture Involving 25–50% of the lobe
V	Laceration Vascular	Involving more than 50% of the lobe Juxta hepatic veins, main hepatic veins or retro hepatic area
VI	Vascular	Hepatic avulsion

Table 2.
American Association for the Surgery of Trauma (AAST) liver injury scale.

If there is a decrease in blood pressure or hematocrit values or the development of any signs of peritonitis, the patient should be immediately taken up for laparotomy.

NOM can be used for penetrating liver trauma in hemodynamically stable patients without peritonitis, significant free air, localized thickened bowel wall, evisceration, and impalement [2, 3].

5.2 Operative management (OM) of traumatic liver injury

Patients should undergo operative management (OM) for liver trauma (blunt and penetrating) in case of hemodynamic instability and concomitant internal organ injury. The primary intention is to control hemorrhage and bile leakage. Major hepatic resections should be avoided in emergency situations and should be considered in subsequent management. Intraoperative management [2, 4] includes:

- hepatic manual compression and hepatic packing
- usage of energy sources such as bipolar cautery, argon laser beams, and so on
- ligation of vessels in the wound
- hepatic debridement
- balloon tamponade
- shunting procedures
- hepatic vascular isolation

For patients undergoing hepatic packing, temporary abdominal closure can be performed to prevent abdominal compartment syndrome. Selective hepatic artery ligation can be considered for patients with massive hemorrhage. Associated portal vein injuries should be repaired because portal vein ligation can lead to hepatic necrosis and bowel edema. Hepatic resections can be performed for severe injuries with uncontrolled bleeding that is not controlled by any of the aforementioned means.

6. Pancreatic injury

Most pancreatic injuries are associated with spinal fracture at the level of the first and second lumbar vertebrae. Isolated injuries of the pancreas after blunt abdominal trauma were noted in 20% of pancreatic injuries. Pancreatic head injuries may be associated with injuries to the stomach, duodenum, and transverse colon. Injuries of the body and tail of the pancreas may be associated with injuries to the stomach, transverse colon, splenic flexure of the colon, splenic vessels, and spleen.

6.1 Clinical presentation

Direct blowing with compression of the upper abdomen against the spine is the most common cause of pancreatic injury. Many patients have minimal clinical symptoms and signs when evaluated after trauma. Pancreatic injuries will be missed if not properly looked for because of minimal symptoms and signs. When symptoms present, the most common is deep epigastric pain associated with nausea and vomiting. Hyperamylasemia is not a precise marker for pancreatic injury. Hyperamylasemia is present in 30–40% of patients admitted with trauma, and the progressive rise in the amylase level over the first 24–48 h of hospitalization is strongly suggestive of pancreatic injury. CECT using 128 slice scanners is the diagnostic modality of choice. Endoscopic retrograde cholangiopancreatography (ERCP) can be used to rule out injury to the main pancreatic duct.

6.2 CT findings

In patients with suspicious pancreatic injuries, CT findings may include:

- fluid in the lesser sac
- fluid between pancreas and splenic vein
- hematoma of transverse mesocolon
- thickening of left anterior renal fascia
- duodenal hematoma or laceration injury to spleen, left kidney, or left adrenal gland
- chance fracture of lumbar spine

CT findings that are diagnostic of pancreatic injuries include:

- parenchymal hematoma or laceration
- obvious transection of the parenchyma
- disruption of head of pancreas
- diffuse swelling characteristics of posttraumatic pancreatitis (**Table 3**) [5]

6.3 Management of isolated pancreatic injuries

In hemodynamically stable patients, pancreatic contusions (AAST grade I), minor capsular injuries, and traumatic pancreatitis can be treated without drainage [6]. Most other injuries require some sort of drainage.

Grade	Type of injury	Description
I	Hematoma Laceration	Minor contusion without duct injury Superficial laceration without duct injury
II	Hematoma Laceration	Major contusion without duct injury or tissue loss Major laceration without duct or injury or tissue loss
III	Laceration	Distal transection or parenchymal injury with duct injury
IV	Laceration	Proximal transection or parenchymal injury involving ampulla
V	Laceration	Massive disruption of pancreatic head

Table 3.
American Association for the Surgery of Trauma (AAST) pancreas injury scale.

AAST grade I injuries are managed with observation and omental pancreatorrhaphy with simple external drainage. Grade II injuries are managed with simple external drainage or omental pancreatorrhaphy and drainage. Grade III injuries are managed with distal pancreatectomy with or without splenectomy, and Roux-en-Y distal pancreatojejunostomy. Grade IV injuries are managed with pancreatoduodenectomy, Roux-en-Y distal pancreatojejunostomy, anterior Roux-en-Y pancreatojejunostomy, and endoscopically placed stent and simple drainage in damage control situations. Grades V and VI injuries are managed with pancreatoduodenectomy.

Complication rates after operative treatment of pancreatic injuries range from 26% to 86%. The most common postoperative infectious complication and the leading cause of morbidity in patients with pancreatic injuries is an intra-abdominal abscess. A pancreatic fistula is the most common pancreatic complication after operative repair of a major injury [5, 6].

7. Renal injury

The most common mechanisms that cause renal injury are motor vehicle collisions, falls, vehicle-associated pedestrian accidents, sports, and assault. Frontal impact caused by acceleration of the occupants into the seat belt or steering wheel, or side impact injuries, occur when the vehicle side panel intrudes into the compartment and hits the occupant, causing renal injury. Frontal and side airbags reduce the risk of renal injury by 45.3% and 52.8%, respectively. Sudden deceleration or a crush injury may result in contusion and laceration of the renal parenchyma. Penetrating renal injuries can occur as a result of gunshot or stab wounds. The incidence of urological tract injury following abdominal trauma is approximately 10%. Renal trauma comprises of 1–5% of all traumas.

7.1 Clinical presentation

Patients may present with localized pain, tenderness, or diffuse tenderness. Retroperitoneal bleeding may lead to abdominal distention, ileus, nausea, and vomiting. Features of hypovolemic shock may be present. Ecchymosis may be present over the flank on the affected side. Lower rib fractures or pelvic fractures may be frequently associated with renal injury. A palpable mass may represent a large retroperitoneal hematoma or perhaps urinary extravasation. If the retroperitoneum has been torn, free blood may be noted in the peritoneal cavity, but no palpable mass will be evident. Hematuria may be present [7].

7.2 Investigations

Contrast-enhanced CT is the gold standard for the evaluation of stable patients with renal trauma. The absence of enhancement on contrast administration or the presence of para hilar hematoma suggests renal pedicle injury and makes it difficult to directly visualize renal vein injury. Standard CECT scans may miss collecting system injury, which is best detected by repeating the scan 10–15 min after contrast injection. CT imaging is both sensitive and specific for demonstrating parenchymal lacerations and urinary extravasations, delineating segmental parenchymal infarcts, and determining the size and location of the surrounding retroperitoneal hematoma and/or associated intra-abdominal injury (spleen, liver, pancreas, and bowel). Renal artery occlusion and global renal infarct are noted on CT scans by lack of parenchymal enhancement or a persistent cortical rim sign.

Grade	Description of injury
I	Contusion or non-expanding subcapsular hematoma No laceration
II	Non-expanding peri renal hematoma Cortical laceration <1 cm deep without extravasation
III	Cortical laceration >1 cm deep with extravasation
IV	Laceration through cortico medullary into collecting system Vascular-segmental renal artery or vein injury with contained hematoma or partial vessel laceration or vessel thrombosis
V	Laceration shattered kidney Vascular: renal pedicle or avulsion

Table 4.
American Association for the Surgery of Trauma (AAST) renal injury scale.

The most common indication for arteriography is nonvisualization of a kidney on intra venous pyelogram (IVP) after major blunt renal trauma when CT is not available. It is the test of choice for evaluating renal vein injury (**Table 4**) [8].

7.3 Nonoperative management (NOM) of traumatic renal injury

Stable patients with blunt renal trauma grades I–IV should be managed conservatively with bed rest, prophylactic antibiotics, and continuous monitoring of vital signs until hematuria resolves. Persistent bleeding represents the main indication for renal exploration and reconstruction.

7.4 Operative management (OM) of traumatic renal injury

Indications for operative renal exploration include:

- hemodynamic instability due to renal hemorrhage
- grade V renal injuries in a stable patient
- expanding or pulsatile perirenal hematoma seen at laparotomy for associated injuries [7].

The goal of renal exploration following renal trauma is the control of hemorrhage and renal salvage. Renorrhaphy or partial nephrectomy is used to manage parenchymal laceration. Attempts should be made for watertight closure of the collecting system. Raw areas should be minimized by using renal capsule, omentum, or fibrin glue. Repair of grade V renal injury is rarely successful, and nephrectomy is usually the best option, except in the case of a solitary kidney. The retroperitoneum should be drained following renal exploration.

7.5 Complications

Early complications occur within the first month of injury and can include bleeding, infection, perinephric abscess, sepsis, urinary fistula, hypertension, urinary extravasation, and urinoma. Delayed complications include calculus formation, chronic pyelonephritis, hypertension, arteriovenous fistula, hydronephrosis, and pseudoaneurysms. Peri-nephric abscesses are best managed by percutaneous drainage. Delayed bleeding and arteriovenous fistula are managed by angiographic embolization. Treatment of hypertension is required if it persists and could include medical management, excision of the ischemic parenchymal segment and vascular reconstruction, or total nephrectomy. Urinary extravasation after renal reconstruction often subsides without intervention if ureteral obstruction and infection are not present. Persistent urinary extravasation responds to stent placement or percutaneous drainage.

8. Mesenteric injury

Isolated mesenteric injury is rare. Mesenteric tears occur because of deceleration injuries. The tear in the mesentery may be longitudinal or transverse. Longitudinal tears are more common than transverse tears. Longitudinal tears can occur from the base of the mesentery to the margin of the gut. The tear may be single or multiple. Longitudinal tears can be suture ligated without bowel resection if they do not extend up to the margin of the gut. Longitudinal tears can involve the root of mesentery and superior mesenteric vessels. Transverse tears are dangerous, as they will cause gangrene of the segment of the bowel. Clinically isolated mesenteric injuries present as follows:

- Immediate—due to bleeding. Signs of continuous bleeding, shock, and peritoneal irritation are present, requiring early laparotomy.

- Delayed—due to bowel infarction. Delayed diagnosis of patients leads to intestinal infarction and requires bowel resection. The patient may present between 12 h and 5 days after injury.

- Due to bowel stenosis or adhesion formation. Mesenteric vascular injury may induce chronic ischemia of the corresponding segment of the small bowel, inducing secondary thickening of the bowel wall and intestinal occlusion and may present between 5 and 8 weeks after injury [9].

9. Traumatic retroperitoneal hematoma

Retroperitoneal injury can be due to blunt or penetrating trauma. Blunt trauma is caused by direct energy transfer. A penetrating injury is an injury that directly violates tissue planes.

The retroperitoneum is divided into three zones.

Zone 1 is the central retroperitoneum from the diaphragm superiorly to the bifurcation of the aorta inferiorly. It contains the inferior vena cava, origins of the major renal and visceral vessels, duodenum, and pancreas. Blunt trauma to this region affects the duodenum and the pancreas to a greater extent, with vascular lesions being less frequent. Pancreatic injuries have an incidence that ranges between 1% and 12% of penetrating trauma and 5% of blunt trauma. The most frequent complication is duodenal fistula.

Zone 2 includes both lateral perinephric areas of the upper retroperitoneum from the renal vessels medially to the lateral reflection of the posterior parietal peritoneum of the abdomen (from the diaphragm superiorly to the level of aortic bifurcation inferiorly). Organs contained include adrenal glands, kidneys, renal vessels, ureter, and ascending and descending colon. Renal and adrenal injuries are common in this region.

Zone 3 is inferior to the aortic bifurcation and includes the right and left internal and external iliac arteries and veins, distal ureter, and distal sigmoid colon and rectum. Mostly vascular injuries occur in this region. Iliac vessel injury occurs in this region [10].

9.1 Management of traumatic mesenteric injury

9.1.1 Penetrating injury

Zone 1—Major vessel injury can occur. Exploration must be done.

Zone 2—Selectively explore the kidney for active hemorrhage or an expanding hematoma. The colon is mobilized to rule out retroperitoneal colon injury and the ureters are explored if in proximity to the wound.

Zone 3—Explore as this is likely a major vascular injury.

9.1.2 Blunt injury

Zone 1—Explore, as this is likely a major vascular injury. The most frequent aortic injuries are infrarenal, while vena cava injuries are predominantly adrenal in origin. In the presence of hemodynamic stability and absence of contraindications, conservative management, including angioembolization, should initially be considered.

Zone 2—Conservative treatment is the most widely accepted. Exploration will be done for an expanding hematoma or one that has failed alternative methods of hemorrhage control, such as angioembolization, for the presence of associated injuries or when there is suspicion of ureteral injuries. Do not explore a contained, nonexpanding hematoma [10].

Zone 3—Do not explore and utilize a method for hemorrhage control, such as intraoperative preperitoneal packing or angioembolization. Iliac vessel injuries prevail in importance due to their associated high mortality. Angiography and venous ligation can be done. The management of bone injury is based on a multidisciplinary approach.

Retroperitoneal Haematoma

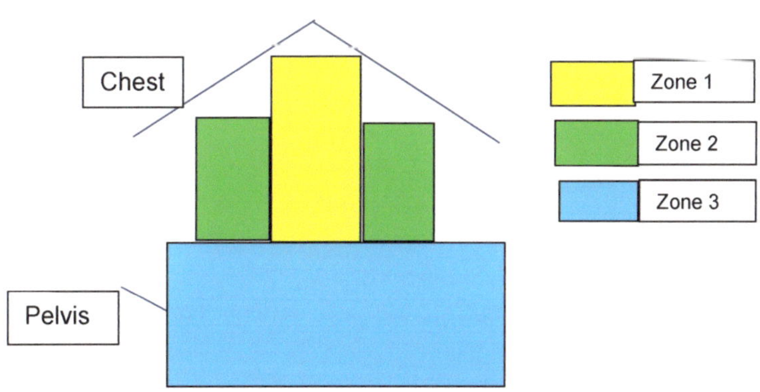

10. Conclusion

Blunt injury of the abdomen is a common abdominal emergency. A high degree of suspicion and watchful screening and examination are needed to diagnose blunt abdominal injury.

Author details

Pabithadevi B. Mehanathan*, Subash Metha, Athisayamani Jeyapaul and Reesha Pa
Department of Surgery, Tirunelveli Medical College, Tirunelveli, Tamilnadu, India

*Address all correspondence to: pabitha73@gmail.com

References

[1] Coccolini F, Fugazzola P, Morganti L, Ceresoli M, Magnone S, Montori G, et al. The World Society of Emergency Surgery (WSES) spleen trauma classification: A useful tool in the management of splenic trauma. World Journal of Emergency Surgery. 2019;**14**(1):1-25

[2] Coccolini F, Catena F, Moore EE, Ivatury R, Biffl W, Peitzman A, et al. WSES classification and guidelines for liver trauma. World Journal of Emergency Surgery [Internet]. 2016;**11**(1):1-8. DOI: 10.1186/s13017-016-0105-2

[3] Stassen NA, Bhullar I, Cheng JD, Crandall M, Friese R, Guillamondegui O, et al. Nonoperative management of blunt hepatic injury: An eastern association for the surgery of trauma practice management guideline. Journal of Trauma and Acute Care. Surgery. 2012;**73**(5 Suppl. 4):20-21

[4] Ahmed N, Vernick JJ. Management of liver trauma in adults. Journal of Emergencies, Trauma, and Shock. 2011 Jan-Mar;**4**(1):114-119

[5] Debi U, Kaur R, Prasad KK, Sinha SK, Sinha A, Singh K. Pancreatic trauma: A concise review. World Journal of Gastroenterology. 2013;**19**(47):9003-9011

[6] Kobayashi L, Kluger Y, Ernest E, Ansaloni L, Biffl W, Leppaniemi A, et al. Duodeno-pancreatic and extrahepatic biliary tree trauma: WSES-AAST guidelines. World Journal of Emergency Surgery. 2019;**15**:1-79

[7] Moore EE, Kluger Y, Biffl W, Leppaniemi A, Matsumura Y, Peitzman AB, et al. Kidney and urotrauma: WSES-AAST guidelines. World Journal of Emergency Surgery. 2019;**14**:1-119

[8] Moore EE, Cogbill TH, Malangoni M, Jurkovich GJ, Champion HR. Scaling system for organ specific injuries. American Association for Surgery of Trauma – Grading for Spleen, Liver, Pancreas and Renal Injuries

[9] Wani I, Bhat RA, Wani S, Khan N, Wani RA, Parray FQ. Isolated small bowel mesentery injury after steering wheel trauma. Trauma Monthly. 2012;**17**(2):279-281

[10] Petrone P, Magadán Álvarez C, Joseph DA, Cartagena L, Ali F, Brathwaite CEM. Approach and management of traumatic retroperitoneal injuries. Cirugia Espanola. 2018;**96**(5):250-259

Chapter 2

Rectus Sheath Hematoma

Serhat Doğan, Selim Sözen, Burhan Hakan Kanat, Gökhan Söğütlü, Mehmet Gençtürk and Hasan Erdem

Abstract

A hematoma is a collection of blood in an extravascular space and is named according to its location. Rectus sheath hematoma (RSH) was first described by Hippocrates and Galen about 25 centuries ago due to abdominal trauma, which is a rare cause of acute abdomen. It is uncommon, which may lead to delayed diagnosis in patients with acute abdomen. This condition arises due to trauma or hypertension in patients with bleeding disorders, using anticoagulants, doing heavy physical exercise, pregnant women, connective tissue diseases, and hematological diseases. The diagnosis can be made by detailed anamnesis, physical examination, ultrasonography, and contrast-enhanced abdominal tomography. For a accurate diagnosis, first of all, the medical history of these patients should be carefully questioned. CT and ultrasonography (USG) are used in the diagnosis of this condition. In many patients, conservative treatment by eliminating the predisposing factor is sufficient. In conclusion, with the increase in use of anticoagulation, the incidence of RSH is expected to increase. Every physician in the surgical field should keep rectus sheath hematoma at the top of the differential diagnosis list in patients presenting with acute abdominal pain and palpable abdominal mass.

Keywords: rectus, sheath, hematoma, trauma, therapy

1. Introduction

A hematoma is a collection of blood in an extravascular space and is named according to its location. Rectus sheath hematoma (RSH) was first described by Hippocrates and Galen about 25 centuries ago due to abdominal trauma. It was the first reported in the modern medical literature by Richardson in 1857 [1, 2].

RSH often has one or more of the risk factors, such as trauma, coagulopathy disorder, obesity, cough, or pregnancy. It may occur due to intense contraction of the rectus muscles during activities associated with the Valsalva maneuver. Patients are usually treated conservatively, but in some cases surgical intervention may be necessary. Cases causing abdominal compartment syndrome requiring surgical or endovascular intervention have been reported in the literature. Today, anticoagulation treatments are applied to more than 6 million patients in the United States for diseases such as atrial fibrillation, mechanical heart valve, or venous thromboembolism. This is a predisposing factor for RSH [3]. Most uncomplicated cases can be managed conservatively. The increasing incidence of RSH also increases the number of complications associated with them. Patients with coagulopathy typically have one of the above-mentioned risk factors, but lack the natural ability to stop bleeding. This ability is also reduced in patients using anticoagulant drugs.

The rectus abdominis muscles originate from the fifth to seventh costal cartilages extend to the pubis, The rectus sheath surrounding the muscle consists of the aponeuroses of the lateral abdominal muscles. The epigastric arteries supply the rectus muscles. The superior epigastric artery is the terminal branch of the internal thoracic artery. The inferior epigastric artery is a branch of the external iliac artery. The inferior epigastric artery runs on the posterior surface of the rectus abdominis and enters the sheath at the arcuate line, passes upward, and anastomoses with the superior epigastric artery. The rectus muscles are separated in the midline by a band of connective tissue called the linea alba.

The rectus sheath is associated with the internal and external oblique muscles from anterior and the fascia of the transversus abdominis muscles from the posterior. Any infection or bleeding that develops in this area can progress through the cellular tissues and can go down to the pelvis. Patients can be taken to emergency operation mostly with the preliminary diagnosis of acute abdomen. Patients without acute abdomen are more stable.

2. Definition

RSH is a clinical condition caused by rupture of the rectus muscle or injury or spontaneous rupture of the epigastric vessels. It is a rare cause of acute abdomen. It is not very common, which may lead to delayed diagnosis in patients with acute abdomen. It can be seen due to trauma or hypertension in patients with bleeding disorders, using anticoagulants, doing heavy physical exercise, pregnant women, connective tissue diseases, and hematological diseases. It can also occur with a sudden sneezing, coughing, or sudden movement. In severe coughing cases, intrathoracic pressures may rise up to 300 mm Hg. With hemodynamic changes, systolic pressure rises up to 140 mmHg in the expiratory phase. These pressure and energy changes can also lead to undesirable results. Cough can cause complications in almost every system, from the cardiovascular system to the musculoskeletal system. RSH may also be one of these complications [4].

3. Clinical presentation

Rectus sheath hematoma has a sudden onset. It usually presents with a palpable mass under the umbilicus in the abdomen. It is more common in elderly patients and women with impaired rectus muscle structure. Pregnancy creates a trauma to the rectus muscle [5]. Ruptures of the superior epigastric artery usually result in small hematomas delimited by the rectus sheath. Hematomas caused by an inferior epigastric artery puncture are larger due to the absence of the posterior rectus sheath below the arcuate line and may grow beyond the midline and posteriorly [6].

Rectus sheath hematomas have abdominal pain in 84–97%, palpable abdominal wall mass in 63–92%, tenderness in 71%, defense in 49%, nausea in 23%, and vomiting and fever in 15%. Patients usually have sharp, severe, and persistent pain. The pain is constant where it does not spread. Pain generally increases with movement [7]. Large hematomas, although rare, can cause urinary tract obstruction and bladder irritability and even abdominal compartment syndrome. If it causes peritoneal irritation, gastrointestinal symptoms such as defense, rebound, tenderness, anorexia, nausea, vomiting, or diarrhea may be present [8]. These findings may be accompanied by weakness, confusion, pallor, and sweating.

Abdominal bruising is a late sign. Bruising in the periumbilical region is a Cullen sign. Bruising in the flank areas is called Grey-Turner's sign. Both symptoms suggest an extraperitoneal extension of the intraperitoneal rupture. An interesting case of a patient with RSH is in the literature due to tetanus. The patient was hemodynamically unstable and was treated with percutaneous arterial embolization. The pathophysiology here is explained as damage to the epigastric arteries due to spasm of the rectus muscle [9].

4. Physical examination

Carnett's sign can help distinguish whether tenderness originates in the abdomen or the abdominal wall. If sensitivity increases or does not change when stretching the abdominal muscles, the test is positive and abdominal wall pathology is more likely. Conversely, in the case of intra-abdominal pathology, tenderness typically decreases when the abdominal muscles contract [10].

Fothergill's sign can help distinguish whether the mass originates in the abdominal wall or inside the abdomen. Fothergill stated that if the mass does not cross the midline and is palpated after contracting the rectus muscles, this is a rectus sheath hematoma [11].

It often occurs in the infraumbilical region and can easily be confused with intra-abdominal inflammation or mass lesions. It is more common in elderly and female patients.

Rectus hematoma has a characteristic appearance. You can easily diagnose it with inspection in the physical examination. For example, our patients photographs are shown in **Figures 1** and **2**.

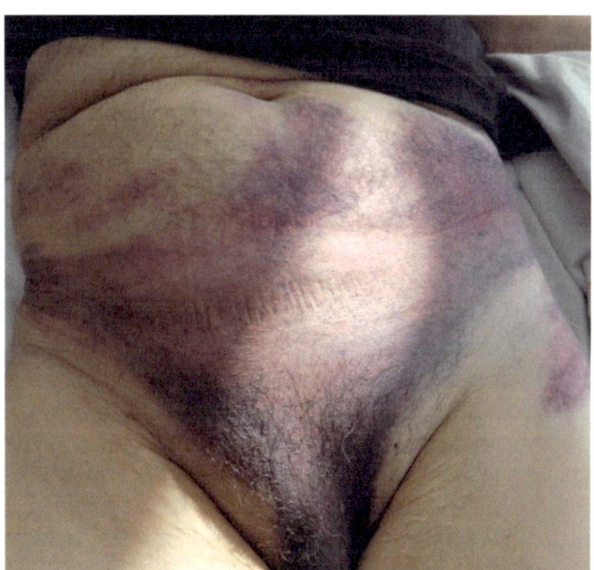

Figure 1.
Photograph of our 77-year-old male patient. One week ago COVID 19 +. He's been hospitalized. He is receiving anticoagulant therapy for coronary artery disease.

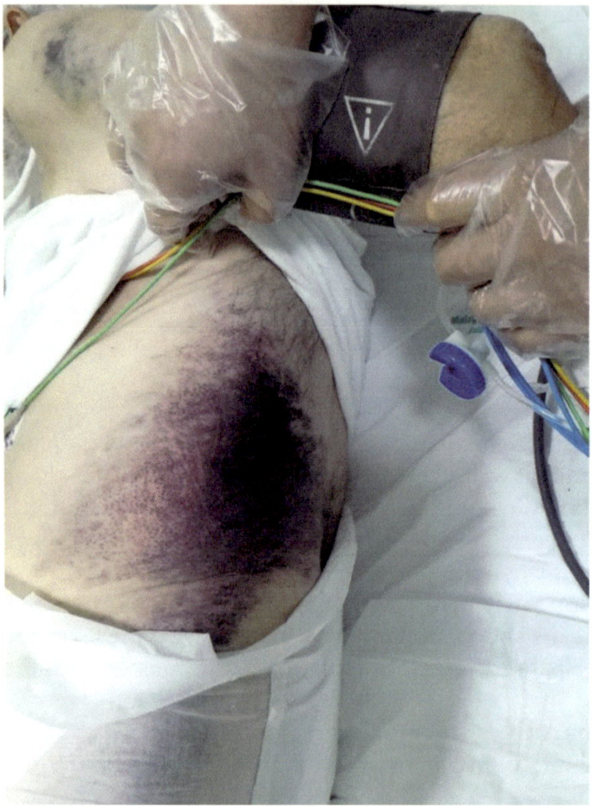

Figure 2.
Photograph of our 86-year-old male patient. He was hospitalized two weeks ago due to COVID 19. At the end of the first week, he was taken to the intensive care unit. He did not use anticoagulants in his anamnesis. He has been receiving subcutaneous low-molecular weight heparin since hospitalization.

5. Diagnosis

The average age of occurrence is 50–60 years [12]. The female male ratio is 2–3/1. It is more common in women [13].

The diagnosis can be made by detailed anamnesis, physical examination, ultrasonography, and contrast-enhanced abdominal tomography. For a correct diagnosis, first of all, the medical history of these patients should be carefully questioned. Drug use should be detailed. CT and ultrasonography (USG) are used in the diagnosis of rectus sheath hematoma. Although USG is used as the first option because it is fast, easy, and quick to reach and can provide information about the location of the mass, CT gives more meaningful results. It should be noted that the sensitivity of ultrasound is 80–90%. Ultrasound may give different results depending on the experience of the attending physician [14]. Tomography can diagnose with sensitivity and specificity reaching 100%. It also allows us to have information about the size, location, origin, spread, and nature of the hematoma. It helps to exclude other abdominal pathologies [15].

In most patients, the hematoma is self-limiting. Complete blood count and bleeding parameters are important in laboratory examinations. They are used for diagnosis and monitoring of treatment. The overall mortality rate in rectus hematoma is 4%. This rate rises to 25% in patients receiving anticoagulation therapy [16].

Treatment of rectus sheath hematoma is evaluated according to its type [17]. Rectus sheath hematomas that develop due to bleeding disorder and do not require intervention are usually limited to close follow-up, rest, and correction of bleeding disorder.

6. Types and treatment approach

It would be beneficial to start the treatment of RSH by first investigating the predisposing factors. After a good anamnesis, most of the predisposing factors are controlled. The drugs used should be carefully examined. Additional diseases of the patient should be evaluated in detail.

Predisposing factors in rectus sheath hematoma are as follows:

1. Trauma.
2. Patients undergoing anticoagulation therapy.
3. Coagulopathy disorder.
4. Cough.
5. Trauma during surgery (iatrogenic).
6. Vascular injury.
7. Severe gagging.
8. Severe vomiting.
9. Severe straining.
10. Obesity.
11. Pregnancy.
12. Tetanus.
13. Heavy physical activity.
14. Sudden sneezing.
15. Hematological diseases.
16. Hypertension.
17. Connective tissue diseases.
18. After sudden movements.

Preventing the predisposing factors mentioned above may be an option in treatment.

RSH is accompanied by many predisposing factors. More than one factor can be present at the same time.

The presence of comorbid diseases, especially in elderly patients, affects the treatment process.

It compels the physician to determine the treatment.

For example, if a patient with heart failure requires transfusion, neither incomplete nor excessive resuscitation should be performed. A balanced policy should be followed.

Or, for example, in a pregnant patient, the treatment protocol should consider the health of the mother and baby.

Rectus sheath hematomas are divided into three types according to their size and localization.

Type I hematoma is within the rectus muscle and only increases the size of the muscle. The hematoma is unilateral and does not spread to the fascia plane. Patients can be followed on an outpatient basis. It can be followed up with bed rest and pain relief. It makes up the majority of patients. It is a limited situation. Close follow-up is important. The course may suddenly worsen, especially in elderly patients.

Type II hematoma can be unilateral or bilateral. Intramuscular hematoma mimics type I, but there is bleeding between the muscle and the transverse fascia. It requires close follow-up due to the possibility of hematoma enlargement. Hospitalization should be given. In this type, rest and analgesics are used. Caution should be exercised in elderly patients. Predisposing factors should be determined and treatment should be planned for it. Frequently hemodynamic monitoring should be performed in the hospital. If necessary, transfusion should be applied. Patients can be discharged within a few days. Hematoma often regresses in 2–4 months (**Figure 3**).

Type III hematoma, bleeding occurs between the muscle and the transverse fascia, in the peritoneum and also to the prevesical area. Patients are hospitalized and treated under close follow-up. Fluid resuscitation and transfusion of blood and blood products may be required in necessary cases. Uncontrolled and progressive hematomas may require surgical intervention.

In such cases, a quick decision must be made. Treatment should be started immediately. Close hemodynamic monitoring is important. In case of teamwork, decisions must be made and implemented quickly. Time is precious and it works fast.

These patients can be discharged after 1 week of follow-up and the hematoma usually resolves in more than 3 months. Rectus sheath hematomas usually do not recur and do not leave sequelae in the long term. The morbidity and mortality rates are higher in receiving anticoagulant therapy, large hematomas, and elderly patients with serious comorbidities [18, 19]. Rapid treatment a bleeding disorder quickly and blood transfusion are the cornerstones of treatment in those receiving anticoagulant therapy.

In many patients, conservative treatment with the elimination of the predisposing factor is sufficient. Correction of coagulation disorders with vitamin K, fresh-frozen plasma, and protamine sulfate and blood replacement are recommended, especially in cases leading to severe anemia. Vascular embolization with catheter, evacuation of hematoma with drainage with USG, or vascular ligation with laparotomy are among the surgical options that can be applied. USG-guided hematoma drainage should always be considered as a minimally invasive option in these patients, as serious complications such as renal failure due to intra-abdominal compartment syndrome and small bowel ischemia may occur due to advanced hematomas (**Table 1**).

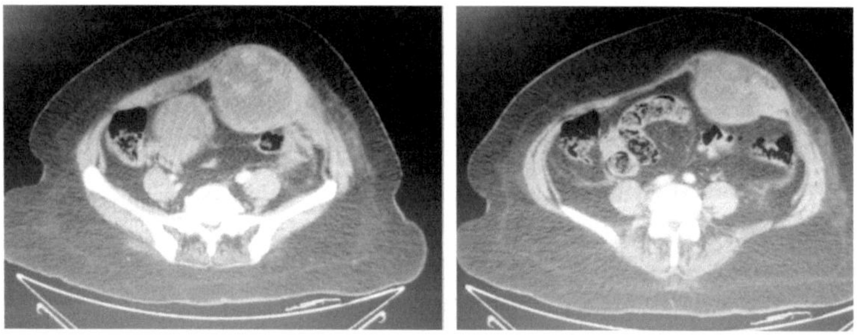

Figure 3.
Rectus sheath hematoma Type II (From Associate Professor Burhan Hakan Kanat's own private archive).

Type	Anatomical extension	Findings	Management
I	Intramuscular, unilateral, no spread to the fascia	No decrease in hemoglobin value	Conservative, outpatient follow-up.
II	Unilateral or bilateral, there is spread to the fascia plane, there is no spread to the prevesical area	Hemoglobin value may decrease	Short-term hospitalization and transfusion may be required
III	There is bilateral spread to the fascia-peritoneum prevesical area	Serious decrease in hemoglobin value and hemodynamic deterioration may be occur	Long-term hospitalization, transfusion with blood and blood products, and surgical intervention may be required

Table 1.
Types of rectus sheath hematomas and principles of clinical approach.

7. Rectus sheat hematoma treatment algorithm

First step Patient → Stabil → Necesseray imaginig analyzes
→ Unstabil → Fast and effective ressusitation

Second Step → Predisposing factors (+) → etiological treatment, eliminating the predisposing factor
→ Predisposing factors (-) → Plan treatment according to the patient condition

Third Step → Classify rectus sheath hematoma as Type I, Type II or Type III

Type I → No decrease in hemoglobin value → Conservative, outpatient follow-up.

Type II → Hemoglobin value may decrease → Short-term hospitalization and transfusion may be required.

Type III → Serious decrease in hemoglobin value and hemodynamic deterioration may be occur → Long-term hospitalization, transfusion with blood and blood products, and surgical intervention may be required

8. Results

In conclusion, with the increasing use of anticoagulation, the incidence of rectus sheath hematoma is expected to increase. Trauma, patients undergoing anticoagulation therapy, coagulopathy disorder, cough, trauma during surgery (iatrogenic), vascular injury, severe gagging, severe vomiting, severe straining, obesity, and many kind of this predisposing factors cause RSH. An effective and fast way of treatment should be followed.

General practitioners, family physicians, emergency physicians, and every physician in the surgical field should keep rectus sheath hematoma at the top of the differential diagnosis list in patients presenting with acute abdominal pain and palpable abdominal mass, especially if there are predisposing factors. Fluid resuscitation or reversal of anticoagulation therapy is of paramount importance. The treatment plan should be decided according to the hemodynamic status of the patient and the characteristics of the hematoma. In the last year, the number of patients using anticoagulants due to COVID-19 has increased and the number of patients diagnosed with rectus sheath hematoma has increased.

Conflict of interest

There is no conflict of interest.

Author details

Serhat Doğan[1*], Selim Sözen[2], Burhan Hakan Kanat[1], Gökhan Söğütlü[1], Mehmet Gençtürk[3] and Hasan Erdem[3]

1 Medical School, Department of General Surgery, Malatya Turgut Özal University, Malatya, Turkey

2 Sözen Surgery Clinic, Department of General Surgery, Vega Hospital, Tekirdağ, Turkey

3 İstanbul Obesity Surgery(IOC) Clinic, Department of General Surgery, Kurtköy Ersoy Hospital, İstanbul, Turkey

*Address all correspondence to: drserhatdogan@gmail.com

References

[1] Manier JW. Rectus sheath hematoma. The American Journal of Gastroenterology. 1972;**57**:443-452

[2] Richardson SB. Rupture of the right rectus abdominis muscle from muscular efforts: Operation and recovery, with remarks. The American Journal of the Medical Sciences. 1857;**33**:41-45

[3] Drinnon K, Simpson SS, Puckett Y, Ronaghan CA, Richmond RE. Rectus sheath hematoma: A rare surgical emergency. Cureus. 2020;**12**(12):e12156. DOI: 10.7759/cureus.12156

[4] Poyraz B, Ülger F. Öksürük Komplikasyonları. Turkiye Klinikleri Journal of Pulmonary Medicine-Special Topics. 2014;**7**(2):10-12

[5] Zengin K, Carkman S, Kiliç I, Beken E, Eyüboğlu E. Treatment approaches to rectus sheath hematoma. Ulus Travma ve Acil Cerrahi Dergisi. 2007;**13**:55-59

[6] Teske JM. Hematoma of the rectus abdominis muscle: Report of a case and analysis of 100 cases from the literatüre. American Journal of Surgery. 1946;**71**: 689-695

[7] Titone C, Lipsius M, Krakauer JS. “Spontaneous” hematoma of the rectus abdominis muscle: Critical review of 50 cases with emphasis on early diagnosis and treatment surgery. Surgery, Original Communication. 1972;**72**(4):568-572

[8] Miyauchi T, Ishikawa M, Miki H. Rectus sheath hematoma in an elderly woman under anti-coagulant therapy. The Journal of Medical Investigation. 2001;**48**(3-4):216-220

[9] Inoue F, Ichiba T, Naitou H. Unusual adverse event of tetanus: Rectus sheath hematoma. Internal Medicine. 2021;**60**(1):151-153. DOI: 10.2169/internalmedicine.4800-20

[10] Carnett JB. Intercostal neuralgia as a cause of abdominal pain and tenderness. Surgery, Gynecology and Obstetrics. 1926;**42**:625-632

[11] Fotherhill WE. Hematoma in the abdominal wall simulating pelvic new growth. British Medical Journal. 1926;**1**: 941-942

[12] Sheth HS, Kumar R, DiNella J, Janov C, Kaldas H, Smith RE. Evaluation of risk factors for rectus sheath hematoma. Clinical and Applied Thrombosis/Hemostasis. 2016;**22**: 292-296

[13] Moreno Gallego A, Aguayo JL, Flores B, Soria T, Hernández Q, Ortiz S, et al. Ultrasonography and computed tomography reduce unnecessary surgery in abdominal rectus sheath haematoma. Journal of British Surgery. 1997;**84**: 1295-1297

[14] Fukuda T, Sakamoto I, Kohzaki S, Uetani M, Mori M, Fujimoto T, et al. Spontaneous rectus sheath hematomas: Clinical and radiological features. Abdominal Imaging. 1996;**21**(1):58-61

[15] Salemis NS, Gourgiotis S, Karalis G. Diagnostic evaluation and management of patients with rectus sheath hematoma. A retrospective study. International Journal of Surgery. 2010;**8**(4):290-293. DOI: 10.1016/j.ijsu.2010.02.011 (Epub 2010 Mar 19)

[16] Donaldson J, Knowles CH, Clark SK, Renfrew I, Lobo MD. Rectus sheath haematoma associated with low molecular weight heparin: A case series. The Annals of The Royal College of Surgeons of England. 2007;**89**:309-312

[17] Berná JD, Garcia-Medina V, Guirao J, Garcia-Medina J. Rectus sheath hematoma: Diagnostic classification by CT. Abdominal Imaging. 1996;**21**:62-64

[18] Ducatman BS, Ludwig J, Hurt RD. Fatal rectus sheath hematoma. JAMA. 1983;**249**:924-925

[19] Dineen RA, Lewis NR, Altaf N. Small bowel infarction complicating rectus sheath haematoma in an anticoagulated patient. Medical Science Monitor. 2005;**11**(10):CS57-CS59

Section 2

Vascular Surgery and Trauma

Chapter 3

Blunt Traumatic Aortic Injury

Domenico Calcaterra

Abstract

Traumatic aortic injuries represent a leading cause of death following motor-vehicular accidents. These injuries curry a very high mortality rate even though a significant number of patients reaches the hospital alive. These injuries are identified in the contest of a polytrauma work up and are almost always associated with multiple other severe traumatic injuries which makes the management of these patients very challenging. The technology advancements seen in recent years with radiologic imaging and the progress of the therapeutic options brought up by the uprise of endovascular therapy, along with the sophistication of the techniques of trauma resuscitation and intensive care management, have improved significantly the overall prognosis of these patients. Although traumatic aortic injuries need to be generally considered a life-threatening condition, their degree of severity may differ significantly from case to case requiring immediate repair in some patients, whereas their repair can be delayed in cases when the severity of the aortic injury does not represent an immediate threat to the patient life. Therefore, the challenge of treatment of the polytrauma patients with an aortic injury is to identify the best strategy of therapy able to prioritize the treatment of the injuries based on their lethal potential. In this contest, the ability of properly defining the severity of the aortic injury is the key-factor to allow the appropriate definition of a treatment strategy able to identify treatment priorities. In our experience, radiologic assessment of the aortic injury in correlation with the evaluation of clinical parameters and a comprehensive polytrauma assessment allows to optimize the ability of the trauma team to establish the most appropriate strategy for the care of this complex patients' group.

Keywords: polytrauma assessment, traumatic aortic injury, thoracic endovascular aortic repair, radiologic assessment

1. Introduction

Traumatic aortic injuries (TAI) represent the second leading cause of death from motor vehicle crashes, accounting for 15% of all motor vehicle accident associated deaths [1–3]. According to a historical case series, death occurs at the scene of the accident in 70 to 90% of these cases [1, 3–7], and of the patients (75%) who arrive to the hospital alive, although hemodynamically stable, only 10% survives more than 6 hours [1, 3]. Patients with TAI surviving at the scene who arrive to the hospital alive most frequently present with an injury at the aortic isthmus, since periadventitial tissue in this location seems to provide some degree of protection against free rupture, allowing the necessary time to transfer the patient from the trauma scene to the hospital [8–10]. The majority of patients with BAI have an

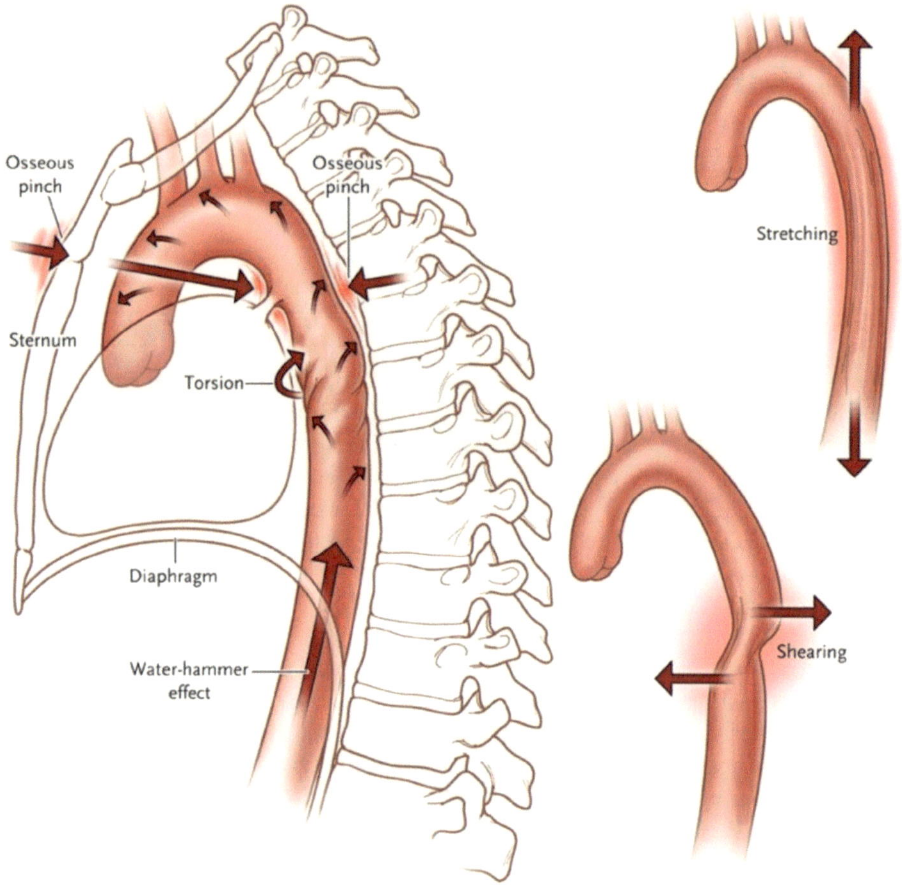

Figure 1.
Theories of blunt aortic injury. Blunt aortic injuries involve a combination of forces, including stretching, shearing, torsion, a "water-hammer" effect (which involves simultaneous occlusion of the aorta and a sudden elevation in blood pressure), and the "osseous pinch" effect from entrapment of the aorta between the anterior chest wall and the vertebral column (modified with permission) [11].

associated closed head injury (51%), multiple rib fractures (46%), lung contusions (38%), or orthopedic injuries (20–35%) [1].

2. Pathophysiology

Blunt traumatic aortic injuries can involve any thoracic aortic segment, including occasionally even the abdominal aorta. The aortic isthmus is by far the most common location, followed by the ascending aorta (10–25%), the aortic arch (10–20%) and the abdominal aorta (5–10%). The theory is that a combination of sudden deceleration, associated to torsion, stretching and sharing forces, and thoracic compression, would cause the aortic injury (**Figure 1**) [11].

3. Clinical management

Diagnosis is made in the contest of the trauma work up as defined by the Advanced Trauma Life Support (ATLS) guidelines. Computed tomography (CT) scan is by far the test of choice to diagnose TAI with a sensitivity and negative predictive value close to 100%. In the very unusual circumstance that CT scan does not provide a definite answer and some doubt on the presence of a TAI remains, which would only occur in the case of a minimal injury, aortic angiogram, eventually with intravascular ultrasound (IVUS), represents the gold-standard to reach a definitive diagnosis. Once diagnosis is made, the severity of the injury assessed by imaging studies and the polytrauma assessment will dictate the treatment strategy [12].

Based on the application of ATLS protocols, treatment of the different trauma injuries will be prioritized based on their acute lethal potential [10]. Exsanguinating hemorrhages from any location and intracranial injury with mass effect take priority of treatment, unless hemodynamic instability obviously related to the imaging finding of an extremely unstable aortic injury would suggest to proceed with immediate endovascular aortic repair. In general, clinical management of the trauma patient arriving to the hospital requires the application of standard measures of trauma resuscitation aiming at establishing the best possible hemodynamic conditions. Once a TAI is diagnosed, anti-impulsive therapy with short-acting beta-blockers should be instituted, if allowed by hemodynamic conditions, to reduce aortic wall-stress. At that point the timing of the aortic repair should be decided based on the radiologic assessment of the aortic injury, the patient's general conditions, accounting in the decision-making process a polytrauma assessment which will allow to determine the sequence of therapeutic interventions offering the best chance of a positive clinical outcome [10].

In fact, although the vast majority of aortic injuries, based on a traditional 'old-school' approach, would represent an indication for therapeutic intervention, there has been more recently a strong school of thoughts proposing a conservative type of management for the type of injuries with a low lethal potential. In these cases, the therapeutic intervention can be delayed or completely aborted, selecting a strategy of radiologic monitoring which would allow to indicate a need for intervention only in cases showing evolution of the aortic injury in a growing pseudo-aneurysm [13–18].

The Society for Vascular Surgery (SVS) has proposed a grading system for TAI intended to rate the degree of severity of the injury (**Figure 2**) [19, 20]. Nevertheless, this grading system has failed to find reliable clinical correlation with risk of aortic rupture and death [15, 19–22], because this classification is qualitative but not quantitative, since can be useful to define the type of injury (intimal laceration versus intramural hematoma, versus pseudoaneurysm, versus free rupture), but does not include parameters to define size and extension of the injury. In our experience of blunt aortic injuries from 3 Level I Trauma Centers in the US from July 2008 to December 2016, we reviewed a total of 76 patients [12]. We analyzed overall mortality and TAI-related mortality (directly caused by the effects of the aortic injury) at 30 days in relation to factors such as: hemodynamic parameters on presentation (SBP, HR and need for vasopressor medications), timing of treatment, injury severity score (ISS) and aortic injury grade as defined by the Society for Vascular Surgery Clinical Practice Guidelines. Aortic injury (AI) grade was dichotomized as stable, grade I-II, and unstable, grade III-IV [12]. Using a new injury scale system, we classified the AI as "Severe" (Radiographic Severe Injury, RSI) when they included findings of [1] total/partial aortic transection (**Figure 3**), [2] active contrast extravasation (**Figure 4**), or [3] the association of 2 of more of the following: contained contrast extravasation >10 mm in bigger dimension, periaortic hematoma and/or mediastinal hematoma with >10 mm thickness, or left pleural effusion (**Figure 5**). We found that mortality caused by the aortic injury was associated with high ISS, SBP < 100, HR ≥ 100, and vasopressors requirement. Also, our

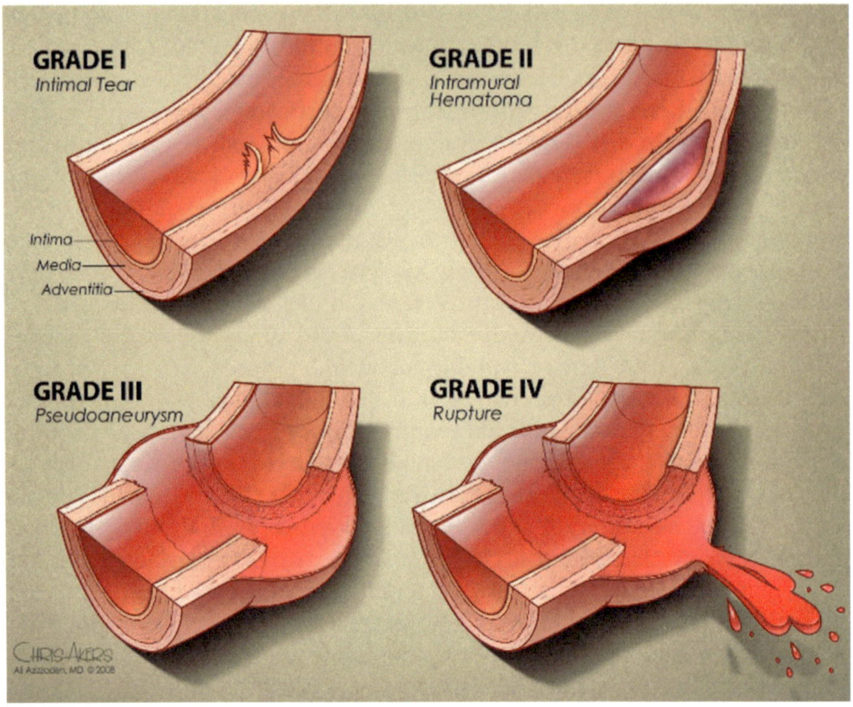

Figure 2.
The Society for Vascular Surgery classification of traumatic aortic injury. Grade I: Intimal tear; grade II: Intramural hematoma; grade III: Pseudoaneurysm; grade IV: Rupture. This grading system has failed to find reliable clinical correlation with risk of aortic rupture and death and therefore cannot find use to indicate the lethal potential of the aortic injury and support the necessary choices that need to be made to select the most appropriate therapeutic strategy to improve the prognosis of the polytrauma patient with TAI (modified with permission) [19].

new classification system of RSI, identifying patients with 'unstable' injuries, found statistically significant association with mortality (**Table 1**).

Therefore, our proposed system of grading of the aortic injury based on radiologic findings and the evaluation of clinical parameters, by the assessment of hemodynamic conditions (SBP, HR, and pressors requirement), is the most important elements to define the severity of the aortic injury and its lethal potential [12].

Besides the exceptional technical advancement of imaging studies that has allowed to increase tremendously the sensitivity to diagnose TAI, the most significant stride in the management of these injuries has been made by the rise of endovascular therapy, since treatment can be delivered with a faster approach using this much less invasive transcatheter technique and with substantial less operative and perioperative risk, compared to the 'open' surgical technique of aorta replacement used as the standard approach until a decade ago [15, 23–25].

Nonetheless, the choice of the most adequate timing for treatment of the aortic injury, particularly with respect to other major traumatic injuries, remains an area of active study. There are currently no clear guidelines for determining which patients may benefit from delayed aortic repair, nor there are validated methods of assessment of the severity of the aortic injury which would allow to choose when prioritize treatment of the aorta [15, 21]. A recent review of a small number of cases has suggested that some patients with small size pseudoaneurysms may be safely managed nonoperatively for the long-term [15, 25, 26]. Nevertheless, the ideal management for stable pseudoaneurysms after BAI remains a subject needing further study.

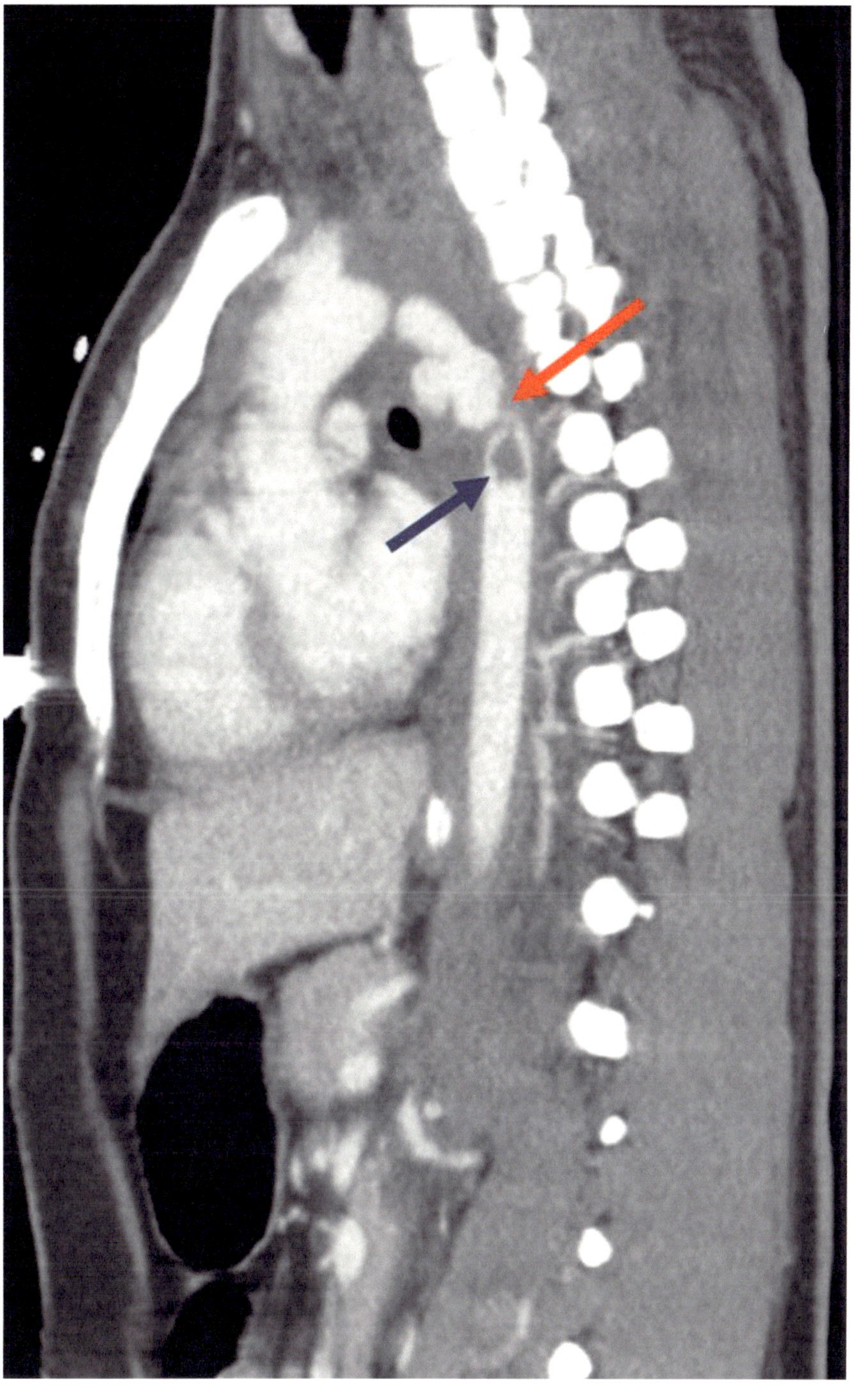

Figure 3.
CT scan of the chest with IV contrast demonstrating aortic transection near the isthmus (red arrow), also associated with intraluminal aortic thrombus as shown by the blue arrow. (transection is defined by total or partial interruption of the column of intra-venous contrast flowing within the aortic lumen).

In this contest, our system of classification created criteria for radiographic assessment of the degree of aortic injury used as a binary variable (severe versus non-severe), allowing to identify the patients in needs for immediate aortic repair.

The standard 'open' surgical technique of repair of TAI has been the replacement of the damaged aortic segment with a synthetic vascular graft. The most common

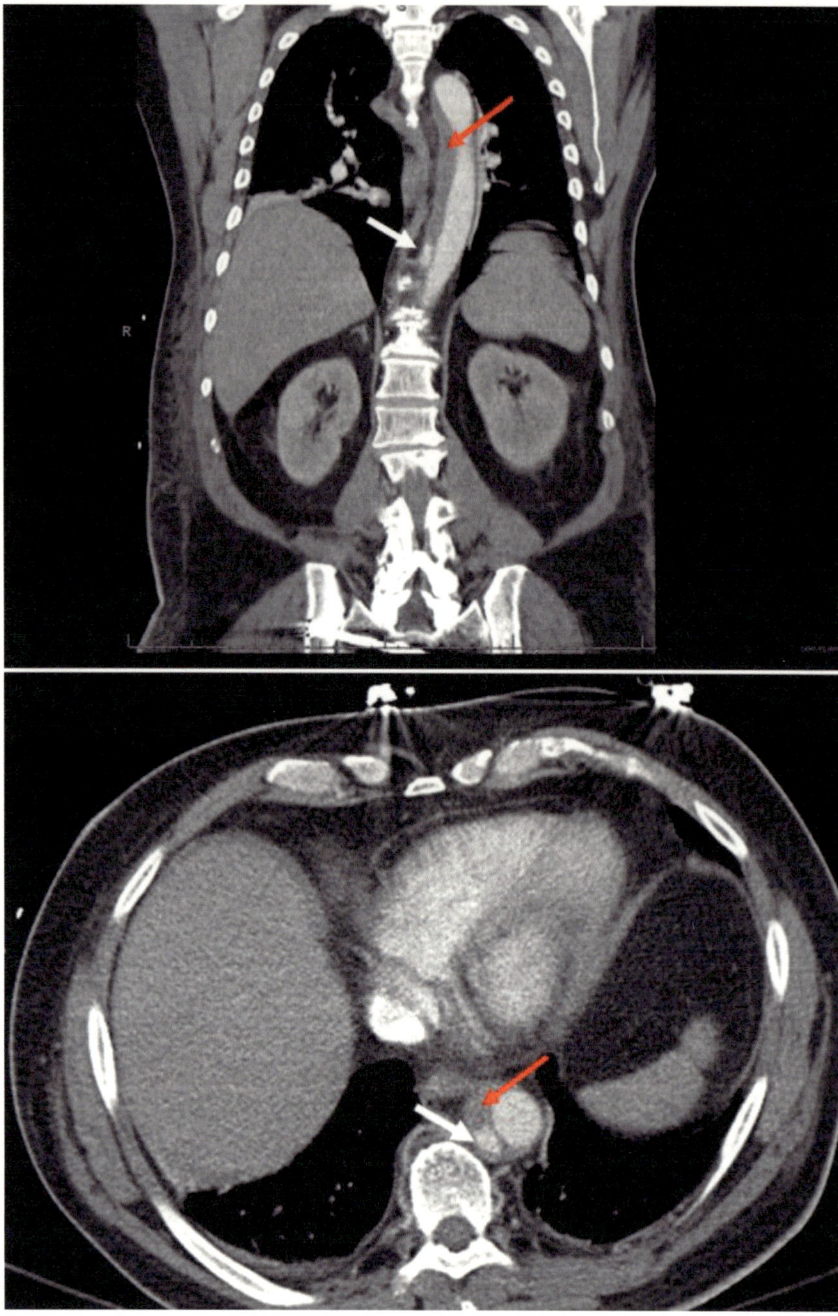

Figure 4.
Sagittal and transverse CT scan images of large intravenous contrast extravasation as shown by red arrows (irregular IV contrast contour outside the aortic wall boundaries).

location of the injury at the aortic isthmus requires a left thoracotomy approach, completing the aortic replacement with left atrial to femoral by-pass (**Figure 6**). This technique had replaced the previous approach of 'clamp and saw' (without use of partial cardiopulmonary bypass), which was associated with a very high incidence of complications, of which paraplegia secondary to spinal cord ischemia was the most common and devastating one. The strategy of replacement using left atrial to femoral bypass allows to maintain perfusion of the lower body after

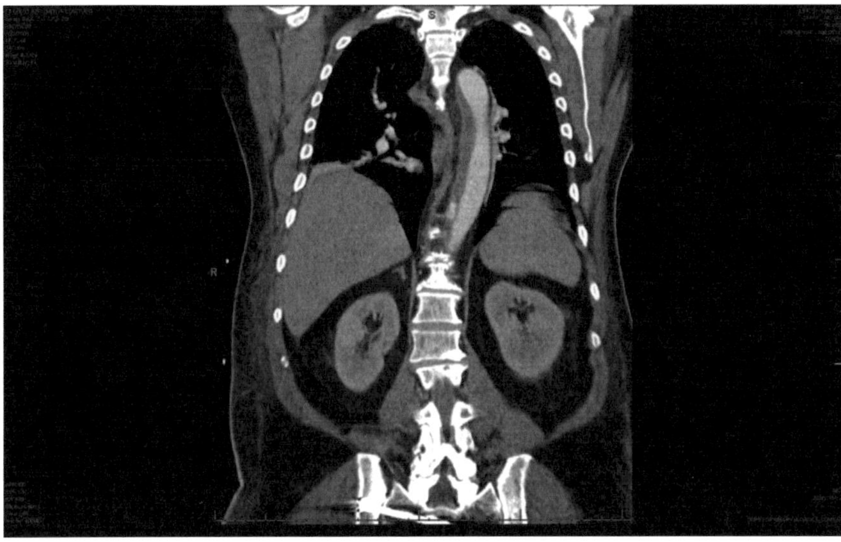

Figure 5.
Coronal and transverse CT scan images of periaortic hematoma (red arrows) and aortic pseudoaneurysm as shown by white arrows (pseudoaneurysm is defined by a regular intravenous contrast contour outside the aortic wall boundaries).

cross-clamping of the aorta above the injured segment, providing a better degree of protection of the spinal cord and other end organs from ischemia (**Figure 6**).

Nonetheless, the operation is still associated with significant morbidity and difficult postoperative recovery, considering that has to be accomplished under the very dangerous conditions of an extreme emergency in patients most likely affected by multiple other traumatic injuries.

The real revolution in the treatment of TAI has been accomplished with the uprise of endovascular aortic repair, which has impacted remarkably on the overall prognosis of these patients allowing to obtain an expedite aortic repair, without the need of an open surgical approach, which translates in much lesser procedural stress, much lesser operative risk, especially in the contest of the common poor general condition of the polytrauma patient, and much easier postprocedural recovery.

The other significant progress in the treatment of TAI has been the realization that under certain conditions the repair of TAI ought to be deferred, prioritizing the treatment of other major concomitant traumatic injuries which represented a more immediate danger for the patient. In a relatively recent prospective multicenter study sponsored by the American Association for the Surgery of Trauma (AAST), the effect of early versus delayed repair was observed in 178 patients admitted with BAI between 2005 and 2007. The study concluded that 'delayed repair of 'stable' blunt thoracic aortic injuries is associated with improved survival [16].

The decision establishing the timing of treatment of TAI should be exclusively based on the characteristics of the injury as seen on CT scan imaging and on the assessment of clinical factors in relation to other associated injuries [15, 21–24]. The Injury Severity Score (ISS) has been used to predict risk of morbidity and mortality associated with blunt trauma since the 1970s. It was demonstrated initially to correlate well with length of stay, need for major surgery, significant disability, and death [27, 28]. ISS does have known limitations, such as more limited applicability to penetrating trauma or other trauma patients in which injuries are localized only to one body area [28]. However, it continues to be a valuable tool used prominently in trauma databases to assign an objective value to traumatic injuries and predict risk for significant morbidity/mortality.

	Unadjusted Mortality		Unadjusted BAI-related mortality	
	OR (CI)	P value[1]	OR (CI)	P value[1]
Age	1.01 (0.98, 1.04)	0.406	1.01 (0.98, 1.04)	0.665
ISS	1.07(1.02, 1.11)	0.003	1.07 (1.02, 1.12)	0.004
SBP < 100	10.54(2.61, 42.65)	<0.001	24.00 (2.84, 203.14)	0.004
HR ≥ 100	4.88 (1.37, 17.44)	0.015	7.48 (1.47, 38.17)	0.016
Pressors	7.S6 (2.12, 29.12)	0.002	6.33 (1.52, 26.33)	0.011
AI grade(SVS)	2.65 (0.67, 10.45)	0.164	6.63 (0.79, 55.41)	0.081
RSI	3.02 (0.92, 9.90)	0.068	5.37 (1.28, 22.90)	0.023
	Adjusted Mortality		Adjusted BAI-related mortality'	
	OR (CI)	P value[2]	OR (CI)	P value[2]
ISS	1.04(1.00, 1.09)	0.074	1.05 (1.00, 1.11)	0.062
SBP < 100	5.54(0.71, 43.47)	0.103	13.16 (0.59, 195.18)	0.061
HR ≥ 100	0.99 (0.14, 6.88)	0.991	1.16 (0.12, 10.74)	0.898
Pressors	1.55 (0.28, 8.66)	0.616	0.77(0.12, 4.96)	0.786
RSI	—		2.51 (0.46, 13.75)	0.290

[1]*Univariate logistic regression.*
[2]*Multivariate logistic regression.*
Abbreviations: AI, aortic injury grade group: BAI, blunt aortic injury CI, 95% confidence interval; HR, heart rate; ISS, injury severity score; OR, odds ratio; RSI, radio graphic severe injury; SBP, systolic blood pressure; SVS, society for vascular surgery.

Table 1.
Logistic regression of factors predicting risk of overall mortality and BAI-related mortality [12].

Thoracic endovascular aortic replacement (TEVAR) offers the advantages of a fast delivery of therapy, preventing a dangerous operation with partial cardiopulmonary bypass or hypothermic circulatory arrest, and less risk of postoperative paraplegia. Furthermore, endovascular therapy can be delivered in the operating room under portable fluoroscopy, offering the tremendous benefit of allowing simultaneous delivery of other therapies for associated life-threatening injuries, such as cranial decompression, transcatheter embolization or exploratory laparotomy, which would be significantly delayed by performing an open surgical aortic repair. The benefit of endovascular therapy is supported by the findings in the literature that have consistently shown substantial advantages of TEVAR over open repair in TAI [15, 29–36]. In our series, open repair was selected only when TEVAR was not feasible, such as in cases with no peripheral aortic access due to presence of intraluminal aortic thrombus, small size of femoral vessels, or presence of a total aortic transection which prevented delivery of endovascular therapy, as seen in the case of **Figure 3**.

As last consideration, in our experience we have observed a relatively small number of patients who died before any treatment was established. If historical series had reported that number to be significant, most recent reports have shown that of the patients surviving BAI at the scene, less than 5% would die of a direct aortic complication after arrival at the hospital [23]. The improvement of the techniques of resuscitation and trauma management, along with a consistent and early application of anti-impulsive therapy have positively impacted on the post-admission hospital mortality [23].

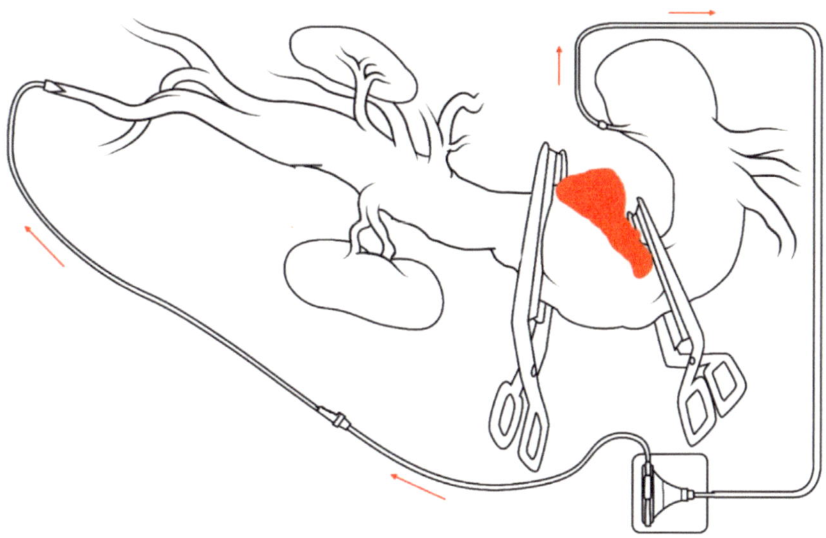

Figure 6.
Technique of proximal descending thoracic aortic replacement with partial cardiopulmonary bypass: Oxygenated blood is drained from the left inferior pulmonary vein and pumped in the left common femoral artery, allowing perfusion of end organs distal to the aortic cross-clamping.

4. Conclusion

The surge of TEVAR as the new standard for treatment for TAI has lowered the operative mortality for the treatment of this condition. However, the optimal timing for the delivery of therapy remains still unclear with respect to the identification of the patients who would require immediate intervention versus the ones for whom postponing treatment of the aortic injury would be preferable. The newly conceived radiologic classification system of TAI we use in our clinical experience is aimed at identifying the type of injuries associated with the highest mortality risk. Radiologic assessment of the severity of the aortic injuries with characterization of the presence of an 'unstable' and life-threatening condition should represent the primary factor to direct management strategy indicating the timing for the aortic repair and guiding treatment priorities.

Author details

Domenico Calcaterra
Florida Atlantic University, Boca Raton, FL, USA

*Address all correspondence to: domenicocalcaterra@hotmail.com

References

[1] Williams, JS, Graff JA, Uku JM, Steinig JP. Aortic injury in vehicular trauma. Ann Thorac Surg. 1994; 57:726.

[2] Razzouk AJ, Gundry SR, Wang N, del Rio MJ, Varnell D, Bailey LL. Repair of traumatic aortic rupture: A 25-year experience. Arch Surg. 2000; 135:913; discussion 919.

[3] Fabian TC, Richardson JD, Croce MA, Smith JS Jr, Rodman G Jr, Kearney PA, Flynn W, Ney AL, Cone JB, Luchette FA, et al. Prospective study of blunt aortic injury: Multicenter Trial of the American Association for the Surgery of Trauma. J Trauma, 1997; 42:374-80: discussion 380-3.

[4] Parmley L, Mattingly T, Manion W. Nonpenetrating traumatic injury of the aorta. Circulation. 1958; 17:1086.

[5] Greendyke RM. Traumatic rupture of aorta; special reference to automobile accidents. JAMA. 1966; 195:527.

[6] Feczko JD, Lynch L, Pless JE, Clark MA, McClain J, Hawley DA. An autopsy case review of 142 nonpenetrating (blunt) injuries of the aorta. J Trauma. 1992; 33:846.

[7] Smith RS, Chang FC. Traumatic rupture of the aorta: Still a lethal injury. Am J Surg. 1986; 152:660.

[8] Arajarvi E, Santavirta S, Tolonen J. Aortic ruptures in seat belt wearers. J Thorac Cardiovasc Surg. 1989; 98:355.

[9] Rabinsky I, Sidhu GS, Wagner RB. Mid-descending aortic traumatic aneurysms. Ann Thorac Surg. 1990; 50:155.

[10] Gleason TG, Bavaria JE. Trauma to the Great Vessels. Cohn LH, ed. Cardiac Surgery in the Adult. New York: McGraw-Hill, 2008:1333-1354.

[11] Neschis DG, Scalea TM, Flinn WR, Griffin BP. Blunt Aortic Injury. N Engl J Med. 2008; 359:1708-1716.

[12] Payne RE, Nygaard RM, Fernandez JD, Sahgal P, Richardson CJ, Bashir M, Parekh K, Vardas PN, Suzuki Y, Corvera J, Krook JC, Calcaterra D. Blunt aortic injuries in the new era: radiologic findings and polytrauma risk assessment dictates management strategy. Eur J Trauma Emerg Surg. 2019 Dec;45(6):951-957.

[13] Symbas PN, Sherman AJ, Silver JM, Symbas JD, Lackey JJ. Traumatic rupture of the aorta. Immediate or delayed repair? Ann Surg. 2002; 235(6):796-802

[14] Estrera AL, Gochnour DC, Azizzadeh A, Miller CC 3rd, Coogan S, Charlton-Ouw K, Holcomb JB, Safi HJ. Progress in the Treatment of Blunt Thoracic Aortic Injury: 12-Year Single-Institution Experience. Ann Thorac Surg. 2010; 90(1):64-71.

[15] Heneghan R, Aarabi S, Quiroga E, Gunn ML, Singh N, Starnes BW. Call for a new classification system and treatment strategy in blunt aortic injury. J Vasc Surg. 2016 Jul;64(1):171-176.

[16] Demetriades D, Velmahos GC, Scalea TM, Jurkovich GJ, Karmy-Jones R, Teixeira PG, Hemmila MR, O'Connor JV, McKenney MO, Moore FO, London J, Singh MJ, Spaniolas K, Keel M, Sugrue M, Wahl WL, Hill J, Wall MJ, Moore EE, Lineen E, Margulies D, Malka V, Chan LS. Blunt traumatic thoracic aortic injuries: early or delayed repair-results of an American Association for the Surgery of Trauma prospective study. J Trauma. 2009 Apr;66(4):967-973.

[17] Nagy K, Fabian T, Rodman G, Fulda G, Rodriguez A, Mirvis S. Guidelines for the diagnosis and

management of blunt aortic injury: An EAST Practice Management Guidelines Work Group. J Trauma. 2000; 48:1128-1143.

[18] Williams MJ, Low CJ, Wilkins GT, Stewart RA. Randomised comparison of the effects of nicardipine and esmolol on coronary artery wall stress: Implications for the risk of plaque rupture. Heart. 2000; 84:377.

[19] Lee WA, Matsumura JS, Mitchell RS, Farber MA, Greenberg RK, Azizzadeh A, Murad MH, Fairman RM. Endovascular repair of traumatic thoracic aortic injury: clinical practice guidelines of the Society for Vascular Surgery. J Vasc Surg. 2011 Jan;53(1):187-192.

[20] Azizzadeh A, Keyhani K, Miller CC 3rd, Coogan SM, Safi HJ, Estrera AL. Blunt traumatic aortic injury: initial experience with endovascular repair. J Vasc Surg. 2009 Jun;49(6):1403-1408.

[21] Fortuna GR Jr, Perlick A, DuBose JJ, Leake SS, Charlton-Ouw KM, Miller CC 3rd, Estrera AL, Azizzadeh A. Injury grade is a predictor of aortic-related death among patients with blunt thoracic aortic injury. J Vasc Surg. 2016 May;63(5):1225-1231.

[22] Lamarche Y, Berger FH, Nicolaou S, Bilawich AM, Louis L, Inacio JR, Janusz MT, Evans D. Vancouver simplified grading system with computed tomographic angiography for blunt aortic injury. J Thorac Cardiovasc Surg. 2012 Aug;144(2):347-354.

[23] Pacini D, Angeli E, Fattori R, Lovato L, Rocchi G, Di Marco L, Bergonzini M, Grillone G, Di Bartolomeo R. Traumatic rupture of the thoracic aorta: ten years of delayed management. J Thorac Cardiovasc Surg. 2005 Apr;129(4):880-884.

[24] Patelis N, Katsargyris A, Klonaris C. Endovascular Repair of Traumatic Isthmic Ruptures: Special Concerns. Front Surg. 2017 Jun 12;4:32.

[25] Tanizaki S, Maeda S, Matano H, Sera M, Nagai H, Nakanishi T, Ishida H. Blunt thoracic aortic injury with small pseudoaneurysm may be managed by nonoperative treatment. J Vasc Surg. 2016 Feb;63(2):341-344.

[26] Osgood M, Heck J, Rellinger E, Doran SL, Garrard CL 3rd, Guzman RJ, Naslund TC, Dattilo JB. Natural history of grade I-II blunt traumatic aortic injury. J Vasc Surg. 2014 Feb;59(2):334-341.

[27] Semmlow JL, Cone R. Utility of the Injury Severity Score: a confirmation. Health Serv Res.1976;11:45-52.

[28] Smith B, Goldberg AJ, Gaughan JP, Seamon MJ. A comparison of Injury Severity Score and New Injury Severity Score after penetrating trauma: A prospective analysis. Journal of Trauma and Acute Care Surgery. 2015;79(2):269-274.26.

[29] Xenos ES, Abedi NN, Davenport DL, Minion DJ, Hamdallah O, Sorial EE, Endean Ed. Meta-analysis of endovascular vs open repair for traumatic descending thoracic aortic rupture. J Vasc Surg. 2008: 48:1343-1351.

[30] Kwolek CJ, Blazick E. Current management of traumatic aortic injuries. Semin Vasc Surg. 2010 Dec;23(4):215-220.

[31] Akowuah E, Baumbach A, Wilde P, Angelini G, Bryan AJ. Emergency repair of traumatic aortic rupture: endovascular versus conventional open repair. J Thorac Cardiovasc Surg. 2007; 134(4):897-901.

[32] Verdant A. Endovascular management of traumatic aortic injuries. Can J Surg. 2006; 49(3):217; author reply 217-218.

[33] Andrassy J, Weidenhagen R, Meimarakis G, Rentsch M, Jauch KW, Kopp R. Stent versus open surgery for acute and chronic traumatic injury of the thoracic aorta: a single-center experience. J Trauma. 2006:60(4):765-771; discussion 771-772.

[34] Kokotsakis J, Kaskarelis I, Misthos P, Athanasiou T, Kanakakis K, Athanasiu C, Romana C, Skouteli E, Lioulias A. Endovascular versus open repair for blunt thoracic aortic injury: short-term results. Ann Thorac Surg. 2007; 84(6):1965-1970.

[35] Akowuah E, Angelini G, Bryan AJ. Open versus endovascular repair of traumatic aortic rupture: a systematic review. J Thorac Cardiovasc Surg. 2009; 138(3):768-769.

[36] Canaud L, Alric P, Branchereau P, Marty-Ané C, Mercier G, Branchereau P. Open versus endovascular repair for patients with acute traumatic rupture of the thoracic aorta. J Thorac Cardiovasc Surg. 2011; 142(5):1032-1037.

Section 3

Chest Trauma

Chapter 4

The Role of Minimally Invasive Surgery in Management of Chest Trauma

Tuba Apaydin

Abstract

The role of minimal invasive surgery in management of chest trauma should not be underestimated. The amount of data for video-assisted thoracoscopic surgery (VATS) management in chest-trauma patient is rare. Nevertheless the on-going acceptance and use of VATS for major thoracic resections has led to advanced techniques for management of major bleedings in the elective-surgery-patient. VATS as a procedure for pleural space management in the non-critical, non-massive-transfusion patients can be of great assistance. Its value in persistent non-major-vessel-bleeding hemothorax in terms of pleural space debridement is unchallenged. In some cases VATS is considered to be related to lower ARDS-rates in comparison to open thoracotomy patients, whereby an obvious bias for the non-massive-injury-patients exist. Jin et al. could prove a significant advantage for stable thoracic trauma patients treated through VATS in a randomised trial vs. open thoracotomy.

Keywords: chest trauma, minimal invasive surgery, video-assisted thoracoscopic surgery

1. Introduction

Video-assisted thoracic surgery (VATS) has a standard role in diagnosis and therapy in thoracic surgery. It has gained a wider spectrum of indications with the improvement in technology and methods. Literature has reported data about its use. Injuries related to the thoracic cage constitutes 25% of mortality in trauma patients. Some of these deaths are ascribable to acute bleeding or cardiac tamponade. However, most of these are because of ARDS, pulmonary contusion, ventilatory associated pnemonia or systemic inflammatory syndrome from empyema or mediastinitis [1].

Patients with chest trauma can be classified in four groups. First group die in the incident or undergo resuscitative thoracotomy in the emergency or operating room due to emergent fatal injuries like cardiac tamponade or acute hemorrage. Secondly, those patients who require emergent thoracotomy for potentially fatal injuries. These patients come to thoracotomy for on-going haemorrage related to non-aortic great vessel, lung parenchymal or chest wall injuries. Also, aortic, oesophageal injuries are in this group. The third group is treated with resuscitation and tube thoracostomy, which is %85 of all chest injured patients. However, retained hemothorax, persistent pneumothorax, on-going haemorrage and empyema will necessitate thoracotomy in %20–30 of these initially non-operatively treated patients. Surgical treatment is also needed for missed injuries of diaphragm, oesophagus and vascular injuries. The fourth group constitutes of patients requiring surgery for complications of hemo- or pneumothoraces or missed injuries [1].

In the past, most patients necessiating surgical treatment secondary to chest trauma was exposed to open thoracotomy, which was the most morbid of surgical incisions. This made way for open thoracotomy as a less invasive method to diagnose and treat thoracic injuries, originally reported by Branco in 1943. The implementation of VATS in trauma was originally reported in a series evaluating diaphragmatic injuries. Afterwards, numerous other indications have been reported [2].

Video-assisted thoracoscopic surgery has become a popular and acceptable method for diagnosis of intra-thoracic lesions since 1990s with the developments in surgical techniques. It is also used for treatment of retained pleural collections, it is a simple alternative to open thoracotomy. Although it's multiple advantages, timing of surgery and its effects on patients' results are not well elucidated. Multiple studies report that prognosis of patients is better with the earlier interventions in injured chest. However, there is so much differences for the optimal time for surgery in these studies [3].

In this chapter, we reported the role of VATS in the management of chest trauma describing characteristics of injury, indications for surgery, methods performed and results in terms of postoperative length of stay, morbidity and mortality [2].

2. Indications of VATS in management of chest trauma

Indications of VATS have been extended for management of diagnosis and treatment of chest trauma since 1990. This approach has multiple advantages as chest tube setting, minimally invasive surgery, less postoperative pain and chest exploration. Today, VATS is used for empyema, persistent pneumothorax, retained haemothorax, mediastinal and diaphragmatic exploration, pleuro-pericardial ruptures, surgery for thoracic duct injury and aspiration of symptomatic foreign bodies. [4].

Persistent pneumothorax is defined as persistent air leak and pneumothorax observed in radiology within 72 hours after chest tube setting. Nearly 23% of pneumothoraces will have a peristent air leak. Several studies reported the effectiveness of VATS in this indication [4–6]. Retained hemothorax is persistent effusion after chest tube insertion on radiographic tools. Retained hemothorax over 300 ml should be an indication for surgery due to its' complications like empyema or pneumonia [7, 8]. 40% of these undrained hemothoraces result in fibrothorax. VATS is also reported that it's useful in the removal of clotted hemothorax. However, procedures performed after 10th. day are hard due to the extensive pleural adhesions.

American Association for the Surgery of Trauma published a significant study related to surgical treatment of retained hemothorax in 328 patients with blunt chest trauma [7]. 33% patients were treated with VATS, 25% required more than two interventions and 5% required more than 3 interventions for complete healing. Thoracotomy for unsuccessful VATS was required in 20% patients. Meyer et al. compared VATS vs. second chest tube setting including 39 patients in each group. VATS diminished duration of chest drainage, duration of hospital stay and hospital costs. Additionally, the second chest tube setting resulted in surgical treatment in 40% patients. VATS should be chosen over second chest tube setting for management of retained hemothorax [9].

Cobanoglu et al. compared chest tube setting vs. VATS as the first intervention for treatment of blunt chest trauma, including 60 patients [10]. VATS decreased duration of hospital stay and the number of reoperations. In the chest tube group, indications for reoperation were clotted hemothorax (23%), empyema (13%), fibrothorax (6%) and continuing bleeding over 100 ml/h (3%). Besides, Smith et al. reported to perform the surgery in 5 days while Vassiliu et al. preffered this duration as 3 days [11, 12]. Nevertheless, Fabrucci et al. reported this duration as the first 48 h for both persistent pneumothorax and retained haemothorax with continuing bleeding over 100 ml/h (**Table 1**) [13].

In haemodynamically stable patients, early VATS should be preferred for retained haemothoraces.

Lazdunski et al. stated that early videotoracoscopic surgery is ideal for management of posttraumatic empyema because it can successfully control the fibrinopurulent phase of empyema and removes the infected hemothorax before the progression of fibrotic phase. However, if the procedure is realised late, a dense fibrotic pleural peel may result with trapped lung at least orient the surgeon to thoracotomy [15].

Traumatic injury to the toracic duct is a rare complication of chest trauma. Videothoracoscopy is a safe and minimally invasive method for ligation of thoracic duct. Lazdunski et al. reported that VATS can be useful for posttraumatic chylothorax if they still exist after 10 days of proper medical therapy and tube thoracostomy [16].

Although most of the patients with chest trauma is treated with chest tube insertion, this conservative method is insufficient in the minority of patients.

Over the last several years, VATS after trauma has been used as the first surgical intervention in hemodynamically stable patients who necessiated urgent thoracic exploration within 24 h after the first presentation.

References	Patients	Design	Outcomes	Key results	
				CT	VATS
Meyer *et al.* (1997) USA [9]	n = 39	RCT	Reoperation	42%	0%
	BCT = 15%		CT duration	4.5	2.53
	Indication: RH		LOS	8.13	5.4*
Schermer *et al.* (1999) USA [6]	n = 39	Prospective cohort study	Reoperation	22.2	0[a]
	BCT = 70%		CT duration	11.8	8.1*
	Indication: PP		LOS	16.5	8.4*
Fabbrucci *et al.* (2008) Italy [13]	n = 81	Retrospective cohort study	Reoperation	0	0
	BCT = 97%		CT duration	5.7	6,3
	Indication: PP, RH		LOS	7	7
DuBose *et al.* (2011) USA [14]	n = 328	Prospective cohort study	Reoperation	35.2	30
	BCT = 49%				
	Indication: RH				
Cobanoğlu U *et al.* (2011) Turkey [10]	n = 60	RCT	Reoperation	50	0
	BCT = 62%		CT duration	7.19	4.84*
	Indication: RH		LOS	7.19	4.84*

RH: retained haemothorax; PP: persistent pneumothorax; BCT: blunt chest trauma.
[a]Eleven patients with persistent air leak were excluded from VATS: 4 due to injuries requiring further ICU stay, 3 due to pneumonia, 2 patients were too small for dual lumen intubation and 2 needed further operations.
**P < 0.05.*

Table 1.
Table of evidence for VATS.

Goodman et al. reported that the use of post-trauma VATS is a safe and effective technique in acutely injured and proper trauma patients including 23 patients in their study [16].

Contraindications for VATS include: Hemodynamic instability, intolerance to lateral decubitus position or single-lung ventilation, suspected injuries to the heart or great vessels and severe adhesions due to prior thoracic interventions [16].

3. Conclusion

Videothoracoscopy is a safe and beneficial diagnostic and therapeutic device as an acute approach to selected patients with chest trauma with no indication for emergent thoracotomy or sternotomy. It is also beneficial in the acute or the retarded approach for patients with blunt chest trauma for treatment of clotted hemothorax, persistent pneumothorax, thoracic empyema, chylothorax and diagnosis of diaphragmatic injuries. However, in cases of suspected pericardial injury, videothoracoscopy should not be considered.

Acknowledgements

No contribution by any other author or no funding declared.

Conflict of interest

The authors declare no conflict of interest.

Author details

Tuba Apaydin
Department of Thoracic Surgery, SBU Istanbul Mehmet Akif Ersoy Thoracic and Cardiovascular Training and Research Hospital, Istanbul, Turkey

*Address all correspondence to: tubaapaydn72@gmail.com

References

[1] Ahmed N, Jones D. Video-assisted thoracic surgery: state of the art in trauma care. Injury. 2004;35(5):479-489. doi: 10.1016/S0020-1383(03)00289-4. PMID: 15081325.

[2] Manlulu AV, Lee TW, Thung KH, Wong R, Yim AP. Current indications and results of VATS in the evaluation and management of hemodynamically stable thoracic injuries. Eur J Cardiothorac Surg. 2004;25(6):1048-1053. doi: 10.1016/j.ejcts.2004.02.017. PMID: 15145008.

[3] H.L. Lin, W.Y. Huang, C. Yang, *et al.* How early should VATS be performed for retained haemothorax in blunt chest trauma? Injury, 2014;45,1359-1364. doi: 10.1016/j.injury.2014.05.036

[4] de Lesquen H, Avaro JP, Gust L. et al. Surgical management for the first 48 h following blunt chest trauma: state of the art (excluding vascular injuries). Interact Cardiovasc Thorac Surg, 2015;20(3):399-408. doi: 10.1093/icvts/ivu397. PMID: 25476459.

[5] Carrillo EH, Schmacht DC, Gable DR, Spain DA, Richardson JD. Thoracoscopy in the management of posttraumatic persistent pneumothorax. J Am Coll Surg, 1998;186:636-639.

[6] Schermer CR, Matteson BD, Demarest GB III, Albrecht RM, Davis VH. A prospective evaluation of video-assisted thoracic surgery for persistent air leak due to trauma. Am J Surg, 1999;177:480-484.

[7] DuBose J, Inaba K, Okoye O et al. Development of posttraumatic empyema in patients with retained hemothorax: results of a prospective, observational AAST study. J Trauma Acute Care Surg, 2012;73:752-757.

[8] Karmy-Jones R, Holevar M, Sullivan RJ, Fleisig A, Jurkovich GJ. Residual hemothorax after chest tube placement correlates with increased risk of empyema following traumatic injury. Can Respir J, 2008;15(5):255-8. doi: 10.1155/2008/918951. PMID; PMCID.

[9] Meyer DM, Jessen ME, Wait MA, Estrera AS. Early evacuation of traumatic retained hemothoraces using thoracoscopy: a prospective, randomized trial. Ann Thorac Surg, 1997;64(5):1396-1400. doi: 10.1016/S0003-4975(97)00899-0. PMID: 9386710.

[10] Cobanoğlu U, Sayir F, Mergan D. Should videothorascopic surgery be the first choice in isolated traumatic hemothorax? A prospective randomized controlled study. Ulus Travma Acil Cerrahi Derg, 2011; 17(2): 117-122. DOI: 10.5505/tjtes.2011.96777

[11] Smith JW, Franklin GA, Harbrecht BG, Richardson JD. Early VATS for blunt chest trauma: a management technique underutilized by acute care surgeons. J Trauma, 2011;71(1):102-105. doi:10.1097/TA.0b013e3182223080. PMID: 21818019.

[12] Vassiliu P, Velmahos GC, Toutouzas KG. Timing, safety, and efficacy of thoracoscopic evacuation of undrained post-traumatic hemothorax, Am Surg. 2001;67(12):1165-1169. PMID: 11768822.

[13] Fabbrucci P, Nocentini L, Secci S. et al. Video-assisted thoracoscopy in the early diagnosis and management of post-traumatic pneumothorax and hemothorax. Surg Endosc. 2008;22(5):1227-1231. doi: 10.1007/s00464-007-9594-0. PMID: 17943365.

[14] DuBose J, Inaba K, Demetriades D et al. AAST Retained Hemothorax Study Group. Management of post-traumatic retained hemothorax: a prospective,

observational, multicenter AAST study. J Trauma Acute Care Surg, 2012;72(1): 11-22. doi: 10.1097/TA.0b013e31824 2e368. PMID: 22310111.

[15] Lang-Lazdunski L, Mouroux J, Pons F. et al. Role of videothoracoscopy in chest trauma. Ann Thorac Surg, 1997;63(2):327-333. doi: 10.1016/ s0003-4975(96)00960-5. PMID: 9033295.

[16] Goodman M, Lewis J, Guitron J. et al. Video-assisted thoracoscopic surgery for acute thoracic trauma. J Emerg Trauma Shock, 2013;6(2):106-109. doi:10.4103/0974-2700.110757.

Chapter 5

Surgical Approach to Rib Fractures

Turkan Dubus

Abstract

Rib fractures due to thorax trauma are one of the issues that mostly concern thoracic surgeons. Treatment for rib fractures is usually conservative. However, in some cases, fractured rib can cause complicated situations and surgical repair is required. Very serious respiratory problems occur in multiple costa fractures. Therefore, many advantages of surgical stabilization of the thorax wall have been reported. Especially shortening mechanical ventilation, decreasing the duration of intensive care unit stay, is important in preventing complications. Operation indications; Persistent pain despite intercostal block, narcotic and nonsteroidal anti-inflammatory analgesics, It was determined upon the presence of leakage from the thorax tube, intrathoracic hematoma and flail chest deformity. Nowadays, nithinol plates and titanium plates are frequently used in surgeon fixation of the rib fractures.

Keywords: Trauma, rib, fracture, surgical fixation, plaque

1. Introduction

The ribs are rigid and flexible structures that make up the chest skeleton and are a set of twelve paired bones. Pain, tenderness, cracking sound with movement in the chest area in cases such as compression, falling, hitting, and beating due to external factors bring to mind the rib fracture. Simple bumps, severe coughing and even sneezing can cause rib fractures in the elderly, where bones are more fragile. It is important to follow up elderly patients with multiple rib fractures in the hospital to prevent complications such as atelectasis and similar complications that may occur in the late period. If the patients are young, uncomplicated rib fractures can be followed up on an outpatient basis. After Blunt trauma rib fractures of incidence is about 30 to 40% [1].

Multiple rib fractures cause severe respiratory problems such as severe pain, dyspnea, flail chest, and atelectasis. Patients need medical or surgical intervention must be made. While the cracks in the ribs caused by traumas are insignificant, rib fractures can lead to intrathoracic organ and vascular injuries. Due to traumas, 4–9. ribs are often affected. 1.-2. fractures in ribs, subclavian vessel and brachial plexus damage, presence of fractures in one or more of the first 3 ribs of the upper thorax, major vascular injuries such as aorta indicate that the trauma is very severe. The fracture point of the ribs is often on the midaxillary line. In fractures in the lower elevations (9th–12th ribs), intraabdominal organ injuries such as liver, spleen and kidney should be investigated. 10–11. ribs fractures are rare because the ribs are more flexible. As the number of rib fractures increases, the risk increases in direct proportion. Complications may vary depending on the localization of rib fractures. Pneumothorax and hemothorax may develop as a result of the sharp end of the broken rib causing lung parenchymal damage, and after tube thoracostomy is applied, rib fractures should be intervened [2].

2. Clinical examination

Pain is the most important symptom indicating rib fracture, and it usually increases with coughing, breathing, and movement. Broken rib ends can be felt with palpation at the time of coughing or deep breathing.

3. Diagnostic methods

3.1 X-ray

It is useful in showing displaced rib fractures, hemothorax and pneumothorax. Almost 50% of rib fractures can be missed on chest radiography. Lateral rib fractures can be hidden by rib lines in the absence of significant separation. Lower rib fractures (10–12th) can be observed on thoracolombar radiographs. Although special radiographs in oblique and bone dose increase the diagnosis rate, it is unnecessary because the treatment will be made according to the clinical findings (**Figure 1**).

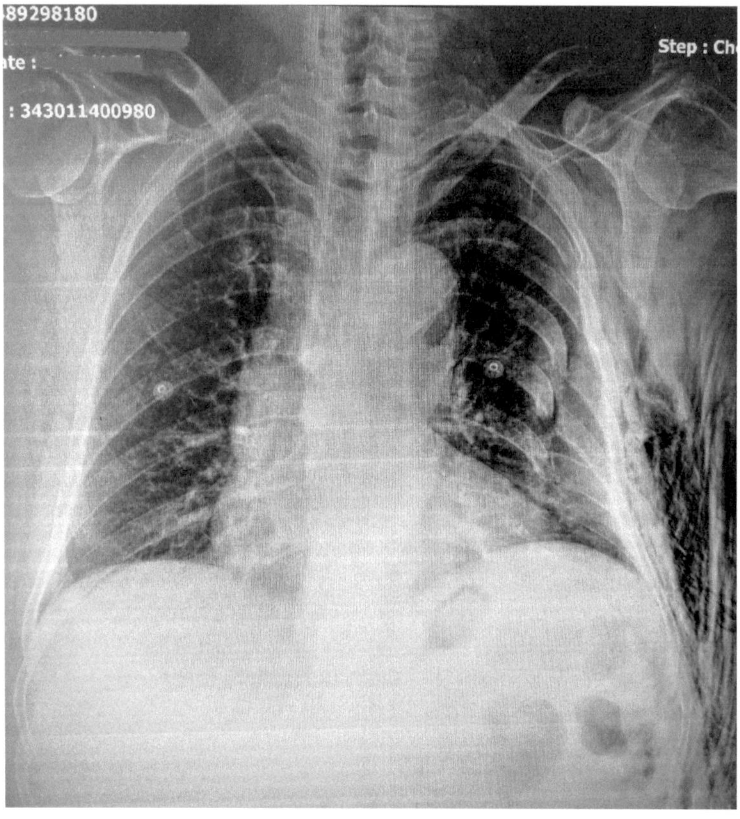

Figure 1.
PA Chest Radiography. Left multiple rib fractures, subcutaneous emphysema.

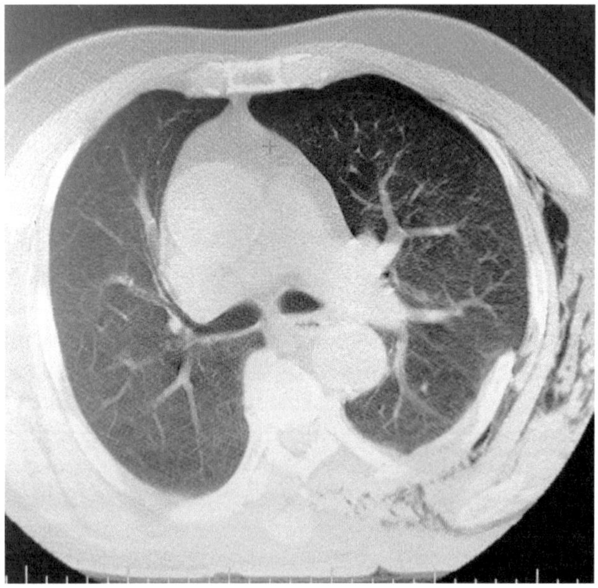

Figure 2.
Computed tomography (CT). Left displaced rib fractures, subcutaneous emphysema and pneumothorax.

3.2 Computed tomography (CT)

It is possible to detect rib fractures, soft tissue and vascular injuries that cannot be detected by x-ray (**Figure 2**).

3.3 Magnetic resonance imaging (MR)

It shows ridge circumference, soft tissue and organ damage. It is also effective in detecting thinner rib fractures.

4. Treatment approaches

4.1 Medical treatment

Most rib fractures, especially nondisplaced ones, heal spontaneously within about six weeks. In medical treatments, epidural catheter application, nonsteroidal anti-inflammatories, intravenous narcotic sedatives and transdermal narcotic agents can be used.

4.2 Nerve blocks

If the pain caused by rib fractures is severe and does not pass, intercostal nerve blockage (long-term anesthesia injection) can be applied.

4.3 Surgical fixation

It is an alternative method to prevent pain and complications due to rib fracture. Surgical intervention is the process of stabilizing the chest wall with rib fixations. Especially patients in intensive care, it plays an important role in reducing the duration of mechanical ventilation and the duration of stay in the intensive care unit, the cost of hospitalization, and the prevention of complications such as infection and morbidity [1].

The flail chest is formed by fractures of at least 3 adjacent ribs in at least 2 different places. Close follow-up of these patients and combating pain and secretions are important. If hypoxia develops in the sail chest, endotracheal intubation and a mechanical ventilator are required in the intensive care unit. With open reduction, rib fixation reduces the morbidity of the patient, and the need for mechanical ventilators and pulmonary infections [3, 4].

The indication for fixation of ribs is usually performing thoracotomy for another reason and applying fixation in this session. The durability of the fixation method to be chosen in the fixation application of the patient is also important. Plate application is very difficult, especially in rib fractures that develop in the posterior. A strong fixation should be provided against breathing, cough and the impacts that may come from outside. Nondisplaced rib fracture ends spontaneously heal by merging with callus formation. However, if the union does not occur at the displaced rib fracture ends, it causes serious pain in the patient (**Table 1**) [4–6].

Cho et al. achieved a successful stabilization using the “bone graft and reconstruction plate” in a patient who had previously undergone stabilization with a kirschner wire but no callus occurred [7]. In a series where fixation is applied to the ribs with the help of an absorbable plate, The application helped the patients to leave the ventilator and even if the application was subjective, it was beneficial [8].

Judet pilates (Toothed plates) (Figure 3a–c)
• Broken lines of ribs should be deperiosteed. • It should be shaped according to the shape of the rib at the level of the broken line. • Requires attention in terms of intercostal neurovascular damage during manipulation.
Locking plates (Figure 4a and **b)**
• Easy to apply • No need to form • It does not require any preliminary preparation such as deperiosteering of the ribs • Relatively wider incision than drilling required
U-Plates (Figure 5a and **b)**
• Judget and Locking record hybrid • Can be applied in a shorter, minimally invasive manner • More durable • Top of ribs since it is applied partially, the incidence of intercostal nerve damage and associated chronic pain is low
Bio-absorbable plates (Figure 6)
• Polylactide absorbable plaque-absorbable suture materials • Expensive • Not easy to apply • Intercostal nerve compression-suture rupture
Intramedullary plates (Figure 7a and **b)**
• Difficulty in placing • Migration, loosening, loss of fixation

Table 1.
Types of plates and properties used in the fixation of rib fractures.

DOI: http://dx.doi.org/10.5772/intechopen.98594

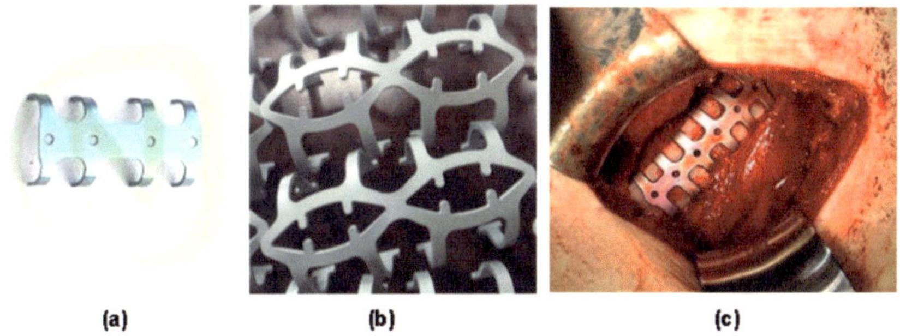

Figure 3.
a–c. Judet plates (toothed plates) and surgical fixation of ribs.

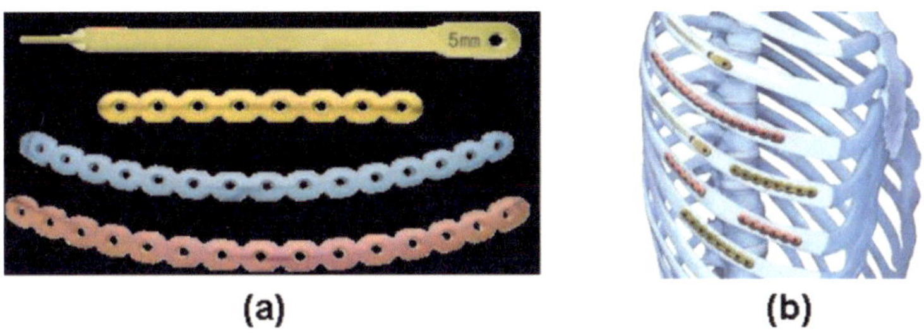

Figure 4.
a and b. Locking plates (locking plates).

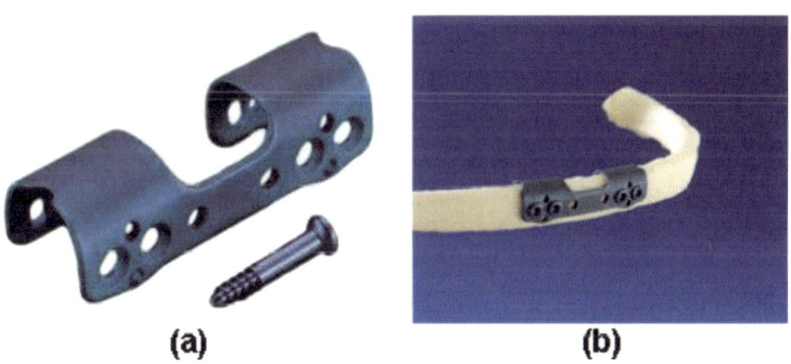

Figure 5.
a and b. U-plates.

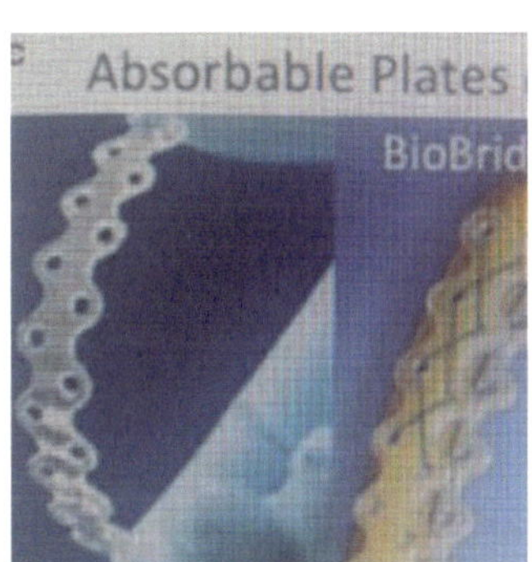

Figure 6.
Bio-absorbable plates.

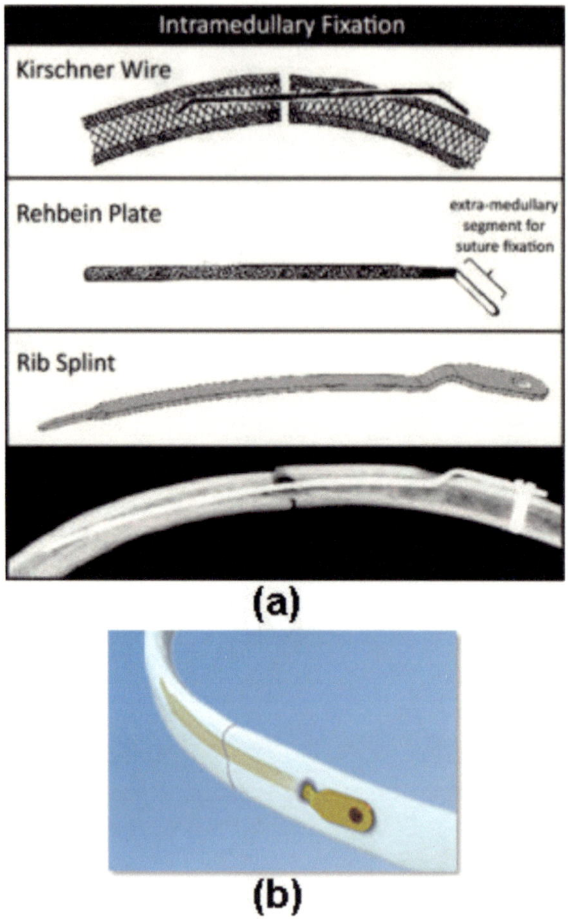

Figure 7.
a and b. Intramedullary plates.

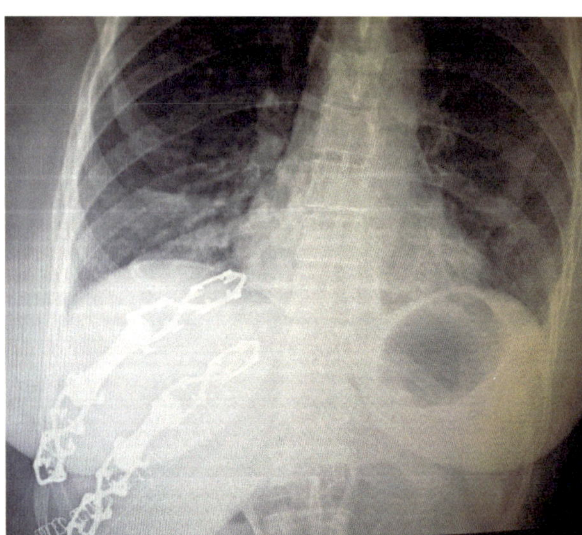

Figure 8.
Chest Radiograpeouhy. Surgical fixation of right rib fractures.

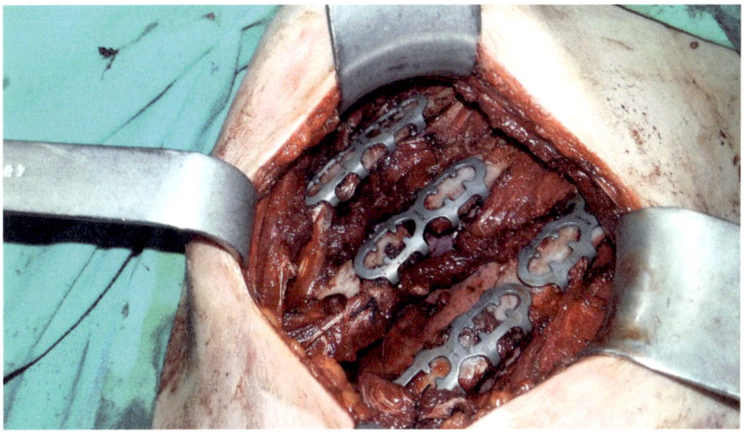

Figure 9.
Use of nithinol plate in rib fractures (Judet plates).

Plaque application is more difficult, especially in rib fractures that develop posteriorly. Researchers who found that intramedullary fixation is both easier and safer in these cases also underlined that the rib splint is more advantageous than the kirschner wire [9]. It is also important that the material to be used in stabilizing the rib fractures does not cause problems in later imaging methods (**Figure 8**).

Balcı et al. preferred titanium plate for this purpose and found that the material did not interfere with the visualization in thoracic CT and MRI taken after the plate application [10].

Today, MRI compatible titanium and nithinol plates are more preferred in rib fracture fixations. Very successful results are obtained in the short and long term follow-up of the patients (**Figure 9**).

5. Conclusion

Surgical stabilization of rib fractures reduces the possible pulmonary complications of patients. It shortens the duration of hospital stay and the time to return to work, improves the quality of life of the patients by physiologically improving their breathing.

Author details

Turkan Dubus
Department of Thoracic Surgery, University of Health Sciences, Istanbul Basaksehir Cam and Sakura City Hospital, Istanbul, Turkey

*Address all correspondence to: drturkandbs@yahoo.com

References

[1] Marasco SF, Martin K, Niggemeyer L, Summerhayes R, Fitzgerald M, Baileyd M. Impact of rib fixation on quality of life after major trauma with multiple rib fractures. Injury. 2019-01-01, Volume 50, Issue 1, Pages 119-124, DOI: 10.1016/j.injury. 2018.11.005

[2] Schuurmans J, Goslings JC, Schepers T. Operative management versus non-operative management of rib fractures in flail chest injuries: a systematic review. Eur J Trauma Emerg Surg. 2017- 43:163-168. DOI: 10.1007/s00068-016-0721-2

[3] Negin Sedaghat N, Chiong C, Tjahjono R, Hsu J. Early Outcomes of Surgical Stabilisation of Traumatic Rib Fractures: Single-Center Review With a Real-World Evidence Perspective. Journal of Surgical Research, 2021-08-01, Volume 264, Pages 222-229. DOI: 10.1016/j.jss.2021.02.026

[4] Beks R, Peek J, de Jong MB, Wessem KJP, Oner CF, Hietbrink F, Leenen LPH, Groenwold RHH, Houwert RM. Fixation of flail chest or multiple rib fractures: current evidence and how to proceed. A systematic review and meta-analysis. Eur J Trauma Emerg Surg. 2019 Aug;45(4):631-644. DOI: 10.1007/s00068-018-1020-x

[5] Zhang, D., Zhou, X., Yang, Y. et al. Minimally invasive surgery rib fracture fixation based on location and anatomical landmarks. Eur J Trauma Emerg Surg 2021. DOI: 10.1007/s00068-021-01676-2

[6] Zhang Q, Song L, Ning S, Xie H, Li N, Wang Y. Recent advances in rib fracture fixation. Journal of Thoracic Disease, Vol 11, Suppl 8 May 2019. DOI: 10.21037/jtd.2019.04.99

[7] de Jonga MB, Houwert RM, van Heerdea S, de Steenwinkel M, F. Hietbrink F, Leenena LPH. Surgical treatment of rib fracture nonunion: A single center experience. Injury, 2018-03-01, Volume 49, Issue 3, Pages 599-603. DOI: 10.1016/j.injury.2018.01.004

[8] Dehghan N. Challenges in plate fixation of chest wall injuries. Injury, 2018-06-01, Volume 49, Pages S39-S43 . DOI: 10.1016/S0020-1383(18)30301-2

[9] Nirula R. Postoperative Complications After Rib Fracture Repair. Rib Fracture. Management, 2018, pp 159-163. https://doi.org/10.1007/978-3-319-91644-6_14

[10] Agababaoglu I, Hasan Ersöz H. The benefits of early rib fixation for clinical outcomes of flail chest patients in intensive care unit. Turkish Journal of Thoracic and Cardiovascular Surgery 2020;28(2):331-339. DOI: 10.5606/tgkdc.dergisi.2020.18439

Section 4

Head Trauma or Traumatic Brain Injury

Chapter 6

Management of Traumatic Brain Injury

Soe Wunna Htay

Abstract

Head trauma or traumatic brain injury (TBI) is one of the most serious, life-threatening conditions in trauma victims. Prompt and appropriate therapy is essential to obtain a favorable outcome. The aim of the acute care of patients with brain injury is to optimize cerebral perfusion and oxygenation and to avoid secondary brain injury. Secondary brain injury develops with times and cause further damage to nervous tissues. The common denominators of secondary injury are cerebral hypoxia and ischemia. A systemic approach such as the Advanced Trauma Life Support (ATLS) algorithm has been recommended for managing head injury patients. Quick initial assessment of the patient's neurologic condition thoroughly is mandatory. There should be attention in evidence of intrathoracic or intraperitoneal hemorrhage in multiple traumatized patients. Optimizing the open airway and adequate ventilation depending on patient's neurologic condition is first step in emergency therapy. Cerebral perfusion pressure should be maintained between 50 and 70 mmHg. Systemic hypotension is one of the major contributors to poor outcome after head trauma. Careful stabilization of the blood pressure with fluid resuscitation and a continuous infusion of an inotrope or vasopressor may be necessary. Standard monitoring with direct arterial blood pressure monitoring and periodical measurement of arterial blood gases, hematocrit, electrolytes, glucose, and serum osmolarity are important. Brain monitoring as with an electroencephalogram, evoked potentials, jugular venous bulb oxygen saturation (Sjo2), flow velocity measured by transcranial Doppler (TCD), brain tissue oxygenation (btPo2), and ICP monitoring may be used. The reduction of elevated ICP by means of giving barbituates, hyperventilation, diuretics and hyperosmolar fluid therapy, body posture and incremental CSF drainage are critical. Seizure prophylaxis, early enteral feeding, stress ulcer prophylaxis, prevention of hyperglycemic state, fever and prophylaxis against deep venous thrombosis in neurointensive care unit are also important after successful resuscitation of head trauma patients.

Keywords: traumatic brain injury, head trauma

1. Introduction

Head trauma or traumatic brain injury (TBI) is one of the most serious, life-threatening clinical problem related with long-term neurobehavioral and socioeconomic consequences in trauma victim [1].

Prompt and appropriate therapy is necessary to obtain a favorable outcome. The management of patient with head injury focuses aggressively on the stabilization and resuscitation of the patient from hypoxia, hypoventilation and cardiovascular collapse. These preventable and treatable secondary insults can complicate the course of patients with head injuries and adversely affect outcome.

2. Systemic and intracranial causes of secondary brain injury

Systemic causes	Intracranial causes
Hypotension	Intracranial hypertension
Hypoxia	Edema
Hypoglycemia/hyperglycemia	Vasospasm
Acidosis	Seizures
Sepsis	Infection
Hyperthermia	
Coagulopathy	
Anemia	

The neurosurgical team members especially anesthesiologists manage perioperative course, taking the patients from the emergency room to the neuroradiology suite, the operating room, and the neurointensive care unit.

3. Emergency management

3.1 Initial assessment of the patient's condition

Glasgow Coma Scale (GCS) assessment can be used for assessing neurologic condition of head trauma patient. Trained health care providers can measure GCS. GCS is based on 15 point scale for estimating severity of brain injury following trauma [2].

1. GCS score of 3 to 8 represents severe head injury.

2. GCS score of 9 to 12 represents moderate injury.

3. GCS score of 13 to 15 represents mild injury [3].

Pupillary responses (size, light reflex) and symmetry of motor function in the extremities should be quickly examined [4].

Head trauma patients are also associated with injury to other parts of body. If the patients presented with shock, thoracic and abdominal injury should be assessed for intrathoracic or intrabdominal bleeding.

3.2 Advanced trauma life support (ATLS) algorithm

There is best accomplished by using a systemic approach, Advanced Trauma Life Support (ATLS) algorithm, which consists of primary and secondary surveys of the patient.

3.2.1 Primary survey

A brief history taking and examination have to be performed within a short period. The history is obtained according to the AMPLE mnemonic (allergies, medications, past medical history, last meal and event). Examination and immediate resuscitation are performed according to the ABCDE mnemonic (airway, breathing, circulation, disability, exposure).

i. Airway management of the patient: The careful monitoring of changes in mean arterial pressure (MAP), intracranial pressure (ICP), and partial pressures of arterial carbon dioxide ($PaCO_2$) and oxygen (PaO_2) during airway management of traumatic brain injury patent is essential.

   Indications for intubation include

   - inability to protect the airway,
   - difficulty with either oxygenation or ventilation,
   - shock,
   - GCS score <9, or
   - Rapid neurologic deterioration [5].

   If the cervical spine injury has not been precluded, manual in line stabilization of head and neck is important during endotracheal intubation. Rapid sequence induction and intubation have to perform in patient with full stomach, using direct laryngoscopy. Flexible fiberoptic intubation may be valuable in patient who have difficult airway and unstable cervical spine fractures. Laryngeal mask airways (LMAs) including the intubating LMAs and surgical airway techniques such as cricothyroidotomy and tracheotomy are useful back up techniques for ventilation and intubation.

   Intravenous uses of lidocaine, 1.5 mg/kg as a pretreatment before endotracheal intubation has been shown to blunt the increase in ICP in response to airway manipulation [6]. If the vital signs of patient are stable, using propofol and thiopental during induction can decrease intracranial pressure and cerebral metabolic rate of oxygen consumption ($CMRO_2$). While hemodynamic condition of the patient is unstable etomidate 0.3 mg/kg may be a better choice [7].

   Use of muscle relaxants facilitate tracheal intubation and decrease the risk of straining. 1 to 1.5 mg/kg of depolarizing muscle relaxant, succinylcholine can be given in emergence condition. Succinylcholine is contraindicated in TBI associated with spinal cord crush, or burn injury owing to the risk of hyperkalemia [8]. Nondepolarizing neuromuscular blocking drugs (NDNMB) including rocuronium, 1 mg/kg, and mivacurium, 0.2 mg/kg, do not increase ICP and can be used in endotracheal intubation in emergence condition. However, nondepolarization muscle relexants use have a slower onset of action (60 to 90 seconds) and caution with allergy using these agents [9].

ii. Breathing considerations include the following: Supplemental high-flow oxygen is provided to all patients to prevent hypoxia (PaO_2 <90 mm Hg) regardless of patient's neurologic condition. Positive pressure ventilation is provided to maintain adequate ventilation and oxygenation [10]. In patients who are hypovolemic, PEEP >10 cm H_2O may reduce CBF. Continuous infusion of sedative and analgesic drugs is beneficial in mechanical ventilated patients for synchronizing of ventilation strategy [11].

iii. Cardiovascular stabilization: Decreasing mean arterial pressure (MAP) of head trauma patient is strongly associated with poor outcome [12]. Hypovolemia is often masked by a relatively stable blood pressure secondary to either sympathetic hyperactivity or the reflex response to increased ICP. Systemic hypotension due to hypovolemic or cardiogenic shock should be identified and controlled or definitively treated (e.g., by the release of tension pneumothorax). Careful stabilization of the blood pressure (systolic blood pressure should be maintained at or above 90 mm Hg) with fluid resuscitation and a continuous infusion of an inotrope or vasopressor may be necessary [13].

iv. Disability: If the condition of the patient is stable, neurologic disability should be performed before giving sedative or neuromuscular blocking agents. Pupillary response and the presence of lateralizing signs and spinal motor and sensory levels are carefully noted.

v. Exposure: Unless the patient in hypothermic, the patient is fully undressed and examined for any other associated injuries.

3.2.2 Secondary survey

Thorough history taking and physical examination, laboratory testing such as metabolic panel, complete blood count, prothrombin time (PT) and partial thromboplastin time (PTT), urinalysis, ethanol level, urine drug screen, and blood type and screen, radiological examination of the whole body should be carried out in secondary survey.

4. Monitoring of patients with traumatic brain injury

4.1 Intracranial pressure (ICP) monitoring

In clinical practice, invasive and non-invasive methods of ICP monitoring are used aiming to determine the optimal cerebral perfusion pressure (CPP). Monitoring of ICP is useful, not only as a guide to therapy, but also for assessing the response to the therapy and determining the prognosis.

Brain Trauma Foundation Guidelines lists the following indications [14]:

1. Moderate to severe head injury patient with normal CT scan

2. Two or more following features are noted in admission:

   Age > 40 years,
   BP < 90 mmHg and
   Unilateral or bilateral motor posturing

4.1.1 Invasive ICP monitoring

Today, the intraventricular catheter remains the gold standard for ICP monitoring, as it measures global ICP [14]. Moreover, the intraparenchymal catheters used for ICP monitoring have integrated as a CSF drainage catheter and catheters that detect parameters, such as brain tissue O_2 partial pressure ($PbtO_2$) and cerebral blood flow (CBF).

4.1.2 Non-invasive ICP monitoring

A non-invasive ICP monitor should be readily available throughout the hospital, be inexpensive, accurate and convenient to use.

i. Brain computed tomography (CT): This is the fastest and the most cost-effective method to evaluate raised ICP and associated pathology. A non-contrast CT head can be ruled out the presence of mass lesions, intracranial bleeding or hydrocephalus, as a cause of intracranial hypertension. Findings suggestive of a raised ICP include cerebral edema, midline shift, compression of basal cisterns and changes in gray-white differentiation [15].

ii. Brain magnetic resonance imaging (MRI): This imaging is costly and time consuming so that it is not first line investigation in acute care setting. MRI can evaluate in detail of soft tissue and cerebral parenchymal lesions, which are not detected on CT scan, e.g. diffuse axonal injury [16].

iii. Transcranial Doppler (TCD) Ultrasonography: TCD can monitor the velocity of blood flow in cerebral arteries indirectly. It is easy to use and can be measured as a bedside procedure. The most commonly used artery is middle cerebral artery (MCA). The flow velocity of the blood causes a phase shift in the specific sound wave frequency emitted and recorded by the probe, whereas the wave frequency is either increased or decreased in correlation with the speed of the blood. The blood flow volume can be determined if the diameter of the vessel is known. Showing of reduced flow volume indicates impairment to cerebral blood flow and indirectly increased ICP. But the accuracy of the technique depends on the experience of the operator [17].

iv. Optic Nerve Sheath Diameter (ONSD): The space between the optic nerve and its sheath is filled with CSF and its pressure equals ICP [18]. Optic nerve sheath diameter can be measured by using a transocular ultrasound in brain trauma patients. The studies proved that ONSD >5–6 mm corresponds to ICP ≥ 20 mmHg [19]. Limitations of its use are patients with chronic ocular disease and malignant hypertension [19]. The ONSD measurement technique is cheap, efficient and non-time consuming, but operator dependent.

v. Tympanic membrane displacement (TMD): It measures transmission ICP to perilymphatic space by the use of communication between subarachnoid space and inner ear through the cochlear aqueduct. An increase in ICP is directly transmitted to the footplate of the stapes, displacing the tympanic membrane. Inwards displacement indicates increased ICP, and outwards normal or low ICP [20]. Nevertheless, this practice is lack of accuracy and has to be reconsidered in clinical practice as in quantitative assessment.

4.1.3 Additional tools in ICP monitoring

i. Brain tissue O_2 partial pressure ($PbtO_2$): Measurement of $PbtO_2$ is invasive means of monitoring regional cerebral oxygen tension by inserting a micro-catheter in the white matter [21]. The method can only measure approximately 15 mm2 of brain tissue around the tip. Normal baseline PbtO2 values range from 25 to 35 mmHg. Current guidelines consider $PbtO_2$ of less than 20 mmHg as threshold to consider intervention [22]. It can be useful in multimodal monitoring in neurocritical care as conjunction with ICP monitor.

ii. Jugular bulb saturation ($SjvO_2$): Measurement of $SjvO_2$ by inserting a catheter placed in the jugular bulb can provide information about cerebral oxygen extraction and adequacy of global cerebral blood flow [17]. SjvO2 distinguishes deficient oxygen supply due to reduced cerebral perfusion (SjvO2 < 50%) from hyperemia (SjvO2 > 80%) because of reduced cerebral oxygen consumption. Increased ICP is mainly associated with reduced SjvO2. It is more difficult to use and less reliable than PbtO2 monitoring [22].

iii. Cerebral microdialysis: Cerebral microdialysis allows bedside monitoring to detect cerebral hypoxemia on a cellular level. The method measures glucose, glutamate, lactate, pyruvate, and glycerol concentrations. An increased in lactate/pyruvate ratio and decreased in brain glucose level is associated with poor outcome after TBI [17]. Microdialysis cannot be used extensively due to its time-consuming maintenance and additional costs [22].

iv. Near infrared spectroscopy (NIRS): NIRS is a noninvasive tool to measure cerebral oxygenation by detecting oxygenated to deoxygenated hemoglobin concentration [21]. There are difficulty to use if there is a scalp swelling [16]. That why the use of NIRS is limited in clinical practice.

v. Continuous electroencephalography (cEEG): The use of cEEG is indicated in detection of convulsive and non-convulsive seizures [23]. Focal slowing of underlying rhythms or global EEG suppression or flat EEG patterns provide information of intracranial hypertension. [16]. cEEG can help predict outcome and titrate treatments throughout giving barbiturates [24].

4.2 Others standard monitoring

Baseline monitoring should include electrocardiography, pulse oximetry, capnography and urine output. Invasive hemodynamic monitorings like invasive arterial pressure measurement and central venous pressure is essential in TBI patients [25]. Some of hemodynamic unstable patients need pulmonary artery catheter placement.

Invasive arterial pressure monitoring permits assessment of beat-to-beat variation in blood pressure and regular arterial blood-gas sampling. Central venous pressure monitoring helps optimization of fluid balance and giving vasoactive drugs and parenteral nutrition. Insertion of a pulmonary artery catheter allows the accurate measurement of pulmonary vascular pressure and calculation of cardiac output. Blood glucose, electrolytes, hematocrit, serum osmolarity and coagulation should be monitored periodically [25].

Insertion of an indwelling urinary catheter facilitates measurement of urinary volume and composition of urine. It helps diagnosis of conditions of altered urinary output associated with TBI such as diabetes insipidus (DI), the syndrome of inappropriate antidiuretic hormone (SIADH) secretion, cerebral salt wasting syndrome and the hyperosmolar state [26].

5. General critical measures

Multiple treatment options exist to treat acute intracranial hypertension. The goal of these therapies is to control ICP to less than 20 mmHg [27] and improving parameters. The most recent TBI guidelines from the Brain Trauma Foundation (BTF) suggest that the ICP goal should be less than 22 mmHg [13].

5.1 Intubation and mechanical ventilation

Early and rapid intubation and mechanical ventilation have to be practiced in moderate to severe head trauma patients [5]. During intubation, adequate depth of sedation and elimination of reflexes such as cough and vomiting should be achieved. Mechanical ventilation should aim at avoiding hypoxemia, hypercapnia and hypocapnia [5]. The usual PCO_2 should be kept at values between 35 and 40 mmHg [27]. Generally positive end expiratory pressure (PEEP) can increase intrathoracic pressure and decrease cerebral venous drainage from superior vena cava [28]. PEEP >15 cmH_2O can be applied safely in patients with acute brain injury as it does not have a clinically significant effect on ICP or CPP [10].

5.2 Blood pressure (BP): CPP optimization

Cerebral perfusion pressure (CPP) is key component in management of traumatic brain injury. Cerebral perfusion pressure is defined as mean arterial pressure (MAP) minus intracranial pressure (i.e., CPP=MAP-ICP) [29]. The recommended goal of CPP per BTF guideline is 50–70 mm Hg [30]. CPP less than normal limit may result in ischemic brain injury [30]. CPP directed therapy is based on theoretical aids that maintaining optimal cerebral blood flow is necessary to meet the metabolic needs of the injured brain [31]. The “Lund therapy” is a therapeutic approach that focuses on the reduction of ICP by decreasing intracranial volumes [32].

Brain trauma foundation guidelines suggest that SBP ≥ 100 mmHg should be maintained for patients 50 to 69 years old or ≥ 110 mmHg for patients 15 to 49 years or > 70 years old to decrease mortality and improve outcomes [13].

Improving outcome of high-risk surgical patients depend on optimizing cardiac output and oxygen delivery guided by goal-directed fluid therapy (GDT) [33]. Crystalloids, colloids and blood components are used for fluid resuscitation and conserving cardiovascular stability to ensure adequate tissue perfusion. Fluid resuscitation should be guided not only by blood pressure but also by urinary output and central venous pressure (CVP) [34]. Hypotension may worse neurologic outcome [35].

0.9% normal saline remains widely used as a resuscitation fluid and remains the fluid of choice for patients with brain injury [36]. Lactated Ringer’s solution is slightly hypotonic relative to plasma. Osmolarity should be frequently checked if large amount of lactate ringer solution is used [37]. Hypoosmolar solutions like 5% dextrose in water increase brain water content and consequently increase ICP. Glucose containing solutions are avoided because hyperglycemia is associated with worsened neurologic outcomes [38].

Large volumes (>500 mL) of 6% hetastarch should not be used because they may cause coagulopathy [39]. Patients who have hemoglobin (Hb) (7-8 mg/dl) may require blood and blood products transfusion to optimize oxygen delivery [40]. By reducing oxygen delivery, anemia may aggravate secondary insult of traumatic brain injury [41].

If the blood pressure and cardiac output cannot be restored through fluid resuscitation, continuous administration of inotropic and vasopressor drugs is necessary. An infusion of either phenylephrine or dopamine is recommended to maintain cerebral perfusion pressure (CPP) [13, 15].

5.3 Body positioning

Elevation of head position 20–30 degree may be helpful in managing ICP [42]. Preventing excessive flexion or rotation of the neck, avoiding restrictive neck taping, and minimizing stimuli that could induce cough and Valsalva responses and uses of lignocaine during endotracheal suctioning are important in management of intracranial hypertension [43].

5.4 Temperature control

It has been shown that patients who develop a body temperature > 37.5°C within the first 72 hours, have significantly worse outcomes determined as Glasgow outcome scale (GOS) 1 or 2 [5, 16, 44]. These include intravenous and enteral antipyretic medications, control of room temperature, and cooling blankets or pads [16].

Although hypothermia (32 to 34°C) decreases cerebral metabolism and may reduce CBF and ICP [19], therapeutic hypothermia does not improve long-term outcome [13, 45]. Serious adverse effects such as hypokalemia, atrial and ventricular arrhythmias, hypotension and coagulopathy may be associated with hypothermia [16].

5.5 Glycemic control

Hyperglycemia is associated with increased mortality in patients with TBI [46]. Target glycemic control between 4.4 to 6.7 mmol/L have been shown shortened hospital stay and improve outcome [47]. Hyperglycemia (> 11.1 mmol/L) is associated with 3.6 fold increased risk of mortality [48].

5.6 Seizure prophylaxis

Post-traumatic seizure (PTS) is a long-recognized and debilitating complication after traumatic brain injury [49, 50]. PTS are classified into immediate PTS (occurring within 24 hours of injury), early PTS (occurring within 7 days after injury), and late PTS (occurring after 7 days of post injury) [51]. Seizures can exacerbate intracranial hypertension by increasing cerebral blood flow corresponding with the need of brain oxygen and glucose [52, 53]. Continuous video recording of Encephalography (EEG) can be used as a diagnosis tools for PTS after TBI [54].

Seizure prophylaxis is recommended during the first week after TBI, particularly in high-risk patients such as those who have GCS scores <10; cortical contusion; depressed skull fracture; subdural, epidural, or intracerebral hematoma; penetrating head trauma; or seizures occurring within the first 24 hours after injury [5, 55]. The Brain Trauma Foundation Guidelines recommended the use of phenytoin in early PTS [16, 56, 57].

5.7 Hyperventilation

Hyperventilation is an effective and rapid method of treating intracranial hypertension. In the setting of intracranial hypertension, the goal of $PaCO_2$ should be lower to 30 mmHg or 25–30 mmHg in extreme cases [13]. Reduction of PCO_2 acutely induces vasoconstriction of cerebral arterioles and a decrease in cerebral blood volume, resulting in ICP reduction [19]. The effect supports within 30 minutes after hyperventilation, but generally lasts less than 24 h, due to buffering capacity of CSF compensations [16].

Both global and regional CBF are markedly decreased within 24 to 48 hours after head trauma [58]. Reduction of CBF in early phase of post injury is significantly associated with poor prognosis. Therefore, hyperventilation may have a role as a temporizing measure for the reduction of elevated ICP [59]. Meanwhile, $SjvO_2$ or $PbtO_2$ measurements can be used to monitor oxygen delivery [45, 59]. Hyperventilation should not be abruptly discontinued but should be tapered slowly over 4–6 h to avoid vasodilatation of cerebral arterioles and rebound increases in ICP [60].

5.8 Hyperosmolar therapy

Hyperosmolar therapy has critical role of medical treatment in acute intracranial hypertension by reducing brain volume. The most commonly used medications are mannitol and hypertonic saline (HS) [45].

Mannitol increase serum osmolality, resulting in an osmotic gradient from interstitial to intravascular space, reduction of cerebral edema and ICP. Mannitol also acts by other mechanisms, such as induction of reflex cerebral arteriolar vasoconstriction, improvement in blood rheology, reduction of CSF formation, and free radicals scavenging. The recommended ICP lowering dose of 20% mannitol is 0.25 to 1 g/kg every 6 hours [61]. Adverse effects of mannitol include acute renal failure, electrolyte disturbances and rebound of existing cerebral edema [62, 63].

Hypertonic saline (HS) is used alternatively to Mannitol and induce induction of reflex cerebral arteriolar vasoconstriction, improved deformability of erythrocytes with enhanced microcirculation, and an anti-inflammatory effect due to reduced adhesion of polymononuclear cells in the cerebral microvasculature [16]. Bolus and repeated doses are required until serum sodium level have been raised above normal (145–155 mEq/L) [64]. Possible adverse effects of HS include rebound cerebral edema, electrolyte disturbances (hypokalemia), congestive heart failure, renal failure, hyperchloremic metabolic acidosis, phlebitis, transient hypotension, hemolysis, osmotic demyelination, subarachnoid bleeding, seizures and muscle twitching [65].

5.9 Sedation and analgesia

Sedation and analgesia are an integral part of medical treatment. Patient-ventilator dyssynchrony and agitation increase intrathoracic pressure, which increase CBV and consequently increase ICP [27]. Ideal sedative drugs should have rapid onset and recovery for a quick neurological assessment, a predictable clearance independent of end organ failure and reducing cerebral blood flow and cerebral metabolic rate of oxygen consumption [11].

Opioids, benzodiazepines, propofol, barbituates and dexmedetomidine can be used to provide the sedation goal. The preferred regime is combination of an opioids such as fentanyl (1–3 μg/kg/hr) or sufentanil (0.1–0.6 μg/kg/hr) to provide analgesia and propofol (0.3–3 mg/kg/hr) for sedation [60]. According to the BTF guidelines, the administration of barbiturates is generally reserved for intracranial hypertension, refractory to maximum standard medical and surgical treatment [57].

Combination of nondepolarizing muscle relaxants and sedatives may be used during posturing, coughing, or agitation in head trauma care. When a neuromuscular blockade is used, EEG should be monitored to rule out convulsive states [66].

5.10 Corticosteroids

Recently, the BTF guidelines do not recommend the use of steroids for improving outcome or reducing ICP in TBI patients [59] because steroids are not effective in cytotoxic edema [60]. Steroid use is only indicated for reducing ICP in abscesses or neoplasms associated with vasogenic edema [60].

5.11 Decompressive craniectomy (DC)

Surgical removal of skull bone in effected side followed by evacuation of hematoma is considered if the patient deteriorating or ICP continues to rise [19]. Prompt removal of an acute subdural, epidural, or large solitary intracerebral hematoma is useful measure in traumatic brain injury treatment [67]. Decompressive craniectomy is risky and adverse effects are common. The complications are weighted against the life-threatening circumstances under which surgery is performed [68].

5.12 Cerebrospinal fluid (CSF) drainage

Procedure of CSF removal via external ventricular drainage device, lumbar drain or serial lumbar puncture is simple and tends to reduce intracranial pressure [16, 19]. Use of CSF drainage during the first 12 hours after injury may be considered in patients with an initial GCS <6 [57]. The major risks of EVD placement and CSF drainage include infection, hemorrhage and herniation [69].

5.13 Other measures

Nutritional support is required to facilitate recovery and should be initiated seventh day of post injury is recommended to improve outcome [57]. Recent guidelines suggest that transgastric jejunal feeding is recommended to reduce the incidence of ventilator associated pneumonia [59].

Proton-pump inhibitors, pantoprazole, 40 mg daily is suggested for stress ulcer prophylasix in critical care settings [70].

Supporting with pneumatic compression devices and use of LMWH or low-dose unfractioned heparin should be initiated as soon as possible for prophylaxis against deep venous thrombosis (DVT) [57]. The benefit of using heparin is considered to outweigh the risk of intracranial hemorrhage.

Author details

Soe Wunna Htay
Department of Anesthesiology and Critical Care, May Myo Military Hospital, Mandalay, Myanmar

*Address all correspondence to: swunnah@gmail.com

References

[1] Stelmasiak, Z., A. Dudkowska-Konopa, and K. Rejdak, Head trauma and neuroprotection. Medical Science Monitor, 2000. 6(2): p. RA426-RA432.

[2] Liew, B., et al., Early management of head injury in adults in primary care. Malaysian family physician: the official journal of the Academy of Family Physicians of Malaysia, 2017. 12(1): p. 22.

[3] Mena, J.H., et al., Effect of the modified Glasgow Coma Scale score criteria for mild traumatic brain injury on mortality prediction: comparing classic and modified Glasgow Coma Scale score model scores of 13. The Journal of trauma, 2011. 71(5): p. 1185.

[4] Aitkenhead, A.R., et al., Smith and Aitkenhead's Textbook of Anaesthesia E-Book: Expert Consult-Online & Print. Neurosurgical Anesthesia. Vol. Sixth Edition. 2013: Elsevier Health Sciences. pp 654-656.

[5] Cottrell, J.E. and W.L. Young, Cottrell and Young's neuroanesthesia. Care of Acutely Unstable Patient. Vol. Fifth Edition. 2016: Elsevier Health Sciences. 161-169.

[6] Lev, R. and P. Rosen, Prophylactic lidocaine use preintubation: a review. The Journal of emergency medicine, 1994. 12(4): p. 499-506.

[7] Turner, B.K., et al., Neuroprotective effects of thiopental, propofol, and etomidate. AANA journal, 2005. 73(4): p. 297.

[8] Muñoz-Martínez, T., et al., Contraindications to succinylcholine in the intensive care unit. A prevalence study. Medicina intensiva, 2014. 39(2): p. 90-96.

[9] Tran, D., et al., Rocuronium vs. succinylcholine for rapid sequence intubation: a Cochrane systematic review. Anaesthesia, 2017. 72(6): p. 765-777.

[10] Videtta, W., et al., Effects of positive end-expiratory pressure on intracranial pressure and cerebral perfusion pressure, in Intracranial Pressure and Brain Biochemical Monitoring. 2002, Springer. p. 93-97.

[11] Peluso, L., B.M. Lopez, and R. Badenes, Sedation in TBI Patients, in Traumatic Brain Injury-Neurobiology, Diagnosis and Treatment. 2019, IntechOpen.

[12] Hutchison, J.S., et al., Impact of hypotension and low cerebral perfusion pressure on outcomes in children treated with hypothermia therapy following severe traumatic brain injury: a post hoc analysis of the Hypothermia Pediatric Head Injury Trial. Developmental neuroscience, 2010. 32(5-6): p. 406-412.

[13] Ragland, J. and K. Lee, Critical care management and monitoring of intracranial pressure. Journal of Neurocritical Care, 2016. 9(2): p. 105-112.

[14] Nag, D.S., et al., Intracranial pressure monitoring: Gold standard and recent innovations. World journal of clinical cases, 2019. 7(13): p. 1535.

[15] Abraham, M. and V. Singhal, Intracranial pressure monitoring. Journal of Neuroanaesthesiology and Critical Care, 2015. 2(03): p. 193-203.

[16] Schizodimos, T., et al., An overview of management of intracranial hypertension in the intensive care unit. Journal of Anesthesia, 2020. 34: p. 741-757.

[17] Ristic, A., R. Sutter, and L.A. Steiner, Current neuromonitoring techniques in critical care. Journal of Neuroanaesthesiology and Critical Care, 2015. 2(02): p. 097-103.

[18] Rajajee, V., et al., Optic nerve ultrasound for the detection of raised intracranial pressure. Neurocritical care, 2011. 15(3): p. 506-515.

[19] Sadoughi, A., I. Rybinnik, and R. Cohen, Measurement and management of increased intracranial pressure. The Open Critical Care Medicine Journal, 2013. 6(1).

[20] Gwer, S., et al., The tympanic membrane displacement analyser for monitoring intracranial pressure in children. Child's Nervous System, 2013. 29(6): p. 927-933.

[21] Tasneem, N., et al., Brain multimodality monitoring: a new tool in neurocritical care of comatose patients. Critical care research and practice, 2017. 2017.

[22] Le Roux, P., et al., Consensus summary statement of the international multidisciplinary consensus conference on multimodality monitoring in neurocritical care. Neurocritical care, 2014. 21(2): p. 1-26.

[23] Kurtz, P., K.A. Hanafy, and J. Claassen, Continuous EEG monitoring: is it ready for prime time? Current opinion in critical care, 2009. 15(2): p. 99-109.

[24] Peacock, S.H. and A.D. Tomlinson, Multimodal neuromonitoring in neurocritical care. AACN advanced critical care, 2018. 29(2): p. 183-194.

[25] Frost, E.A., Essentials of Neuroanesthesia and Neurointensive Care. Anesthesia and Analgesia, 2009. 108(2): p. 678-679.

[26] Capatina, C., et al., Diabetes insipidus after traumatic brain injury. Journal of clinical medicine, 2015. 4(7): p. 1448-1462.

[27] Godoy, D.A., S. Lubillo, and A.A. Rabinstein, Pathophysiology and management of intracranial hypertension and tissular brain hypoxia after severe traumatic brain injury: an integrative approach. Neurosurgery Clinics, 2018. 29(2): p. 195-212.

[28] Frost, E.A., Effects of positive end-expiratory pressure on intracranial pressure and compliance in brain-injured patients. Journal of neurosurgery, 1977. 47(2): p. 195-200.

[29] Robertson, C.S., Management of cerebral perfusion pressure after traumatic brain injury. The Journal of the American Society of Anesthesiologists, 2001. 95(6): p. 1513-1517.

[30] Smith, M., Cerebral perfusion pressure, in BJA: British Journal of Anaesthesia. 2015, Oxford University Press: Lhttps://doi.org/10.1093/bja/aev230ondon. p. Pages 488-490.

[31] Prabhakar, H., et al., Current concepts of optimal cerebral perfusion pressure in traumatic brain injury. Journal of anaesthesiology, clinical pharmacology, 2014. 30(3): p. 318.

[32] Nordström, C.-H., Physiological and biochemical principles underlying volume-targeted therapy—the "Lund concept". Neurocritical care, 2005. 2(1): p. 83-95.

[33] Alvis-Miranda, H.R., S.M. Castellar-Leones, and L.R. Moscote-Salazar, Intravenous fluid therapy in traumatic brain injury and decompressive craniectomy. Bulletin of Emergency and Trauma, 2014. 2(1): p. 3.

[34] De Backer, D. and J.-L. Vincent, Should we measure the central venous pressure to guide fluid management? Ten answers to 10 questions. Critical Care, 2018. 22(1): p. 1-6.

[35] Zornow, M.H. and D.S. Prough, Fluid management in patients with traumatic brain injury. New Horiz, 1995. 3(3): p. 488-98.

[36] Alvis-Miranda, H.R., et al., Fluid therapy in neurotrauma: basic and clinical concepts. Reviews in Health Care, 2014. 5(1): p. 7-22.

[37] Thompson, M., et al., Comparison of crystalloid resuscitation fluids for treatment of acute brain injury: a clinical and pre-clinical systematic review and network meta-analysis protocol. Systematic reviews, 2018. 7(1): p. 1-7.

[38] Zornow, M. and D. Prough, Fluid management in patients with traumatic brain injury. New horizons (Baltimore, Md.), 1995. 3(3): p. 488-498.

[39] Kozek-Langenecker, S.A., Effects of hydroxyethyl starch solutions on hemostasis. The Journal of the American Society of Anesthesiologists, 2005. 103(3): p. 654-660.

[40] Badenes, R., et al., Hemoglobin concentrations and RBC transfusion thresholds in patients with acute brain injury: an international survey. Critical care, 2017. 21(1): p. 1-10.

[41] Lelubre, C., et al., Anemia management after acute brain injury. Critical care, 2016. 20(1): p. 1-11.

[42] Schulz-Stübner, S. and R. Thiex, Raising the head-of-bed by 30 degrees reduces ICP and improves CPP without compromising cardiac output in euvolemic patients with traumatic brain injury and subarachnoid haemorrhage: a practice audit. European Journal of Anaesthesiology (EJA), 2006. 23(2): p. 177-180.

[43] Gholamzadeh, S., et al., Examination of the effect of lidocaine on intracranial pressure during endotracheal suctioning in severe head-injured patients in Shiraz-Iran: P 089. European Journal of Anaesthesiology| EJA, 2008. 25: p. 31.

[44] Greer, D.M., et al., Impact of fever on outcome in patients with stroke and neurologic injury: a comprehensive meta-analysis. Stroke, 2008. 39(11): p. 3029-3035.

[45] Stocchetti, N. and A.I. Maas, Traumatic intracranial hypertension. New England Journal of Medicine, 2014. 370(22): p. 2121-2130.

[46] Shi, J., et al., Traumatic brain injury and hyperglycemia, a potentially modifiable risk factor. Oncotarget, 2016. 7(43): p. 71052.

[47] Hermanides, J., et al., Glycaemic control targets after traumatic brain injury: a systematic review and meta-analysis. Critical Care, 2018. 22(1): p. 1-11.

[48] Griesdale, D.E., et al., Glucose control and mortality in patients with severe traumatic brain injury. Neurocritical care, 2009. 11(3): p. 311.

[49] Evans, R.W. and S.C. Schachter, Post-traumatic seizures and epilepsy. UptoDate. Available from: https://www.uptodate.com/contents/post-traumatic-seizures-and-epilepsy, 2014.

[50] Pingue, V., C. Mele, and A. Nardone, Post-traumatic seizures and antiepileptic therapy as predictors of the functional outcome in patients with traumatic brain injury. Scientific reports, 2021. 11(1): p. 1-12.

[51] Nichol, H., J. Boyd, and J. Trier, Seizure Prophylaxis Following Moderate

to Severe Traumatic Brain Injury: Retrospective Investigation of Clinical Practice and the Impact of Clinical Guidelines. Cureus, 2020. 12(4).

[52] Marguc, K., et al., Measurements of CBF in Patients with Epilepsy, in Cerebral Blood Flow and Metabolism Measurement. 1985, Springer. p. 202-204.

[53] Posner, J.B., F. Plum, and A. Van Poznak, Cerebral metabolism during electrically induced seizures in man. Archives of Neurology, 1969. 20(4): p. 388-395.

[54] Piccenna, L., G. Shears, and T.J. O'Brien, Management of post-traumatic epilepsy: An evidence review over the last 5 years and future directions. Epilepsia open, 2017. 2(2): p. 123-144.

[55] Ding, K., P.K. Gupta, and R. Diaz-Arrastia, Epilepsy after traumatic brain injury. Translational research in traumatic brain injury, 2016.

[56] Fordington, S. and M. Manford, A review of seizures and epilepsy following traumatic brain injury. Journal of neurology, 2020. 267: p. 3105-3111.

[57] Carney, N., et al., Guidelines for the management of severe traumatic brain injury. Neurosurgery, 2017. 80(1): p. 6-15.

[58] Stocchetti, N., et al., Hyperventilation in head injury. Chest, 2005. 127(5): p. 1812-1827.

[59] Bullock, M. and J. Povlishock, Brain Trauma Foundation, American Association of Neurological Surgeons, Congress of Neurological Surgeons, AANS/CNS Joint Section on Neurotrauma and Critical Care. Guidelines for the management of severe traumatic brain injury. J Neurotrauma, 2007. 24(suppl 1): p. S1-106.

[60] Mayer, S.A. and J.Y. Chong, Critical care management of increased intracranial pressure. Journal of Intensive Care Medicine, 2002. 17(2): p. 55-67.

[61] Shawkat, H., M.-M. Westwood, and A. Mortimer, Mannitol: a review of its clinical uses. Continuing education in anaesthesia, critical care and pain, 2012. 12(2): p. 82-85.

[62] Shi, J., et al., Hypertonic saline and mannitol in patients with traumatic brain injury: A systematic and meta-analysis. Medicine, 2020. 99(35).

[63] Schwimmbeck, F., et al., Hypertonic saline versus mannitol for traumatic brain injury: a systematic review and meta-analysis with trial sequential analysis. Journal of neurosurgical anesthesiology, 2021. 33(1): p. 10-20.

[64] Ennis, K.M. and G.M. Brophy, Management of intracranial hypertension: Focus on pharmacologic strategies. AACN advanced critical care, 2011. 22(3): p. 177-182.

[65] Georgiadis, A.L. and J.I. Suarez, Hypertonic saline for cerebral edema. Current neurology and neuroscience reports, 2003. 3(6): p. 524-530.

[66] Shapiro, H.M., Intracranial hypertension: therapeutic and anesthetic considerations. The Journal of the American Society of Anesthesiologists, 1975. 43(4): p. 445-471.

[67] Nakagawa, K. and W.S. Smith, Evaluation and management of increased intracranial pressure. CONTINUUM: Lifelong Learning in Neurology, 2011. 17(5): p. 1077-1093.

[68] Stiver, S.I., Complications of decompressive craniectomy for traumatic brain injury. Neurosurgical focus, 2009. 26(6): p. E7.

[69] Grady, M.S., Lumbar drainage for increased intracranial pressure. Journal of neurosurgery, 2009. 110(6): p. 1198-1199.

[70] Ye, Z., et al., Gastrointestinal bleeding prophylaxis for critically ill patients: a clinical practice guideline. Bmj, 2020. 368.

Section 5

Acute Compartment Syndrome

Chapter 7

Acute Compartment Syndrome of the Extremities and Paraspinal Muscles

Balaji Zacharia and Raj Vignesh Selvaraj

Abstract

Acute compartment syndrome (ACS) occurs when the pressure within the closed osteo-fascial compartment raises above perfusion pressure leading to irreversible tissue ischemia and necrosis. Any closed compartment in the body can be affected by ACS. The leg is the commonest site. Trauma is the common cause of compartment syndrome in young patients. In older patients, medical causes can cause it. The diagnosis in a conscious patient can be made based on clinical features. Pain out of proportion to the injury is the most important symptom. Exacerbation of pain on stretching the affected muscles and paresthesia are the common signs. Compartment pressure measurement is important for the diagnosis in unconscious and uncooperative patients. The treatment of established ACS is emergency fasciotomy. Untreated compartment syndrome can lead to neurovascular injuries and muscle contractures. In this chapter, we will see the etiologies, clinical features, investigations, and management of acute compartment syndrome of the extremities and the paraspinal region.

Keywords: acute compartment syndrome, compartment syndrome of extremities, compartment syndrome of paraspinal muscles

1. Introduction

Compartment syndrome is a condition where the pressure within the closed osteo-fascial compartment raises above the perfusion pressure leading to irreversible tissue ischemia and necrosis. A decrease in the compartment volume, an increase in the contents of the compartment, or external pressure can cause it. The compartment syndrome can be acute or chronic. Untreated acute compartment syndrome (ACS) can cause cosmetic problems due to muscle contractures, and functional problems due to neurovascular damages. These can be reasons for litigations against treating doctors. If detected early and treated properly most of the sequelae of ACS are preventable [1]. In 1881 Dr.Richard von Volkmann a German doctor first described ACS [2]. Paul Jepson in 1924 demonstrated ischemic contracture of muscles in animals [10]. The incidence of ACS is 0.7 to 7.3 persons per 100,000 people [3]. The leg is the most common site of ACS. About 2–9% of fractures of the tibia are associated with ACS [4]. There is an equal incidence of ACS in closed and open fractures [5]. A higher incidence of ACS is seen in grade 2 compound fractures than in grade 3A or 3B due to the phenomenon of self-decompression seen in higher grade open injuries. Due to the bulk of muscles attached to the diaphysis of long bones, fractures through

IntechOpen

diaphysis are prone to develop ACS [6]. The forearm, hands, feet, buttocks, thighs, and paraspinal muscles are other sites. Any closed fascial space can be affected [7]. There can be fracture-related and non- fracture-related ACS. Fracture-related ACS is common in young males and its diagnosis is early. Whereas non- fracture-related ACS is common in the elderly with medical comorbidities. The ACS in the elderly can be traumatic or nontraumatic. The posterior compartment of the leg is affected commonly in non-fracture-related ACS group. In older people with swollen limbs, a compartment pressure measurement is needed to rule out ACS [8].

1.1 Etiologies

Most cases of ACS occur following trauma. Young males are about ten times more affected than females. Other than fractures there are many other etiologies. Arterial injuries, snake bite, burns, gunshot injuries, leakage from arterial and venous access, drug overdose, pulsatile lavage, contusions in hemophilia, infection, and intraosseous fluid replacement in infants are other causes for acute compartment syndrome. Over-exertion can lead to acute or chronic compartment syndrome. Lithotomy positioning during surgery or constricting casts or wraps can cause it. ACS can also occur due to non-traumatic medical conditions like nephrotic syndrome, viral myositis, hypothyroidism, bleeding disorders, malignancies, diabetes mellitus (Diabetes –associated muscle infarction), and in rheumatological conditions like ruptured Baker's cyst [9].

An awareness regarding the etiology, pathophysiology, clinical features, investigations and management is essential for all doctors dealing with patients in the emergency department. In this narrative review, we intend to give a detailed overview of acute compartment syndrome.

2. Anatomy of the compartments

The major groups of muscle and neurovascular structures are separated by a thick layer of fascia. The fascia provides a surface for the attachment of muscles and keeps the contour of the muscles. It improves mechanical advantage during contractions. The fascia helps in coordinated actions of muscle and proprioception. These fasciae divide the extremity into different compartments.

There are 4 compartments in the leg. They are anterior, lateral, superficial, and deep posterior compartments. The anterior intermuscular septum separates the lateral muscles from the anterior muscles, and the posterior intermuscular septum separates the lateral muscles from the posterior muscles. The interosseous membrane spans the gap between the tibia and fibula, separating the anterior and deep posterior compartments. The transverse intermuscular septum separates the musculature of the superficial and deep posterior compartments. The anterior compartment contains the anterior tibial artery and veins, deep peroneal nerve. Tibialis anterior, extensor hallucis longus, and extensor digitorum longus are the muscles in this compartment. Peroneus longus and peroneus brevis muscles with superficial peroneal nerves are in the lateral compartment. The superficial posterior compartment contains gastrocnemius, soleus, and plantaris muscles. The peroneal vessels, posterior tibial vessels, tibial nerve and tibials posterior, flexor digitorum longus, and flexor hallucis longus muscles are the contents in the deep posterior compartment of the leg [10].

There are controversies regarding the actual number of compartments in the foot. Various authors reported three to nine compartments in the foot. The medial, lateral, and superficial compartments run along the entire length of the foot. The four interossei and an adductor compartment are confined to the forefoot. Manoli and Weber described a calcaneal compartment containing quadratus Plantae muscle, posterior tibial, and lateral plantar vessels and nerves. The medial compartment contains abductor hallucis brevis, and flexor hallucis brevis, and lateral compartment abductor digiti quinti and flexor digiti quinti. Flexor digitorum brevis and lumbrical muscles in the superficial compartment [11].

The forearm is divided into three compartments volar dorsal and lateral. The interosseus membrane separates the volar and dorsal compartments. The lateral compartment containing the mobile wad muscles is separated by the antebrachial septum is lying in the posterior and lateral part. Volar muscles are commonly affected in ACS. There is anatomical communication between various compartments of the forearm so the release of the volar compartment alone can reduce pressure in others [12]. The thenar, hypothenar, adductor, and interosseous compartments are the main osteo-fascial compartments of the hand [13].

The anterior, medial, and posterior are the fascial compartments in the thigh. The lateral intermuscular septum is very tough whereas the medial and posterior septum is thinner. The hamstrings are in the posterior compartment, adductors in the medial, and quadriceps in the anterior compartments. There is a lot of potential space in the thigh compartments before the elevation of intra compartmental pressure [14].

3. Pathophysiology

ACS is due to elevation of interstitial pressure due to any reason. The difference between interstitial pressure and capillary perfusion pressure (CPP) is the determinant of tissue perfusion. When the volume of an osteo-fascial compartment increases as in intra-compartment bleeding due to injury, both tissue and venous pressure increases. Once this pressure exceeds CPP there is a collapse of capillaries resulting in ischemia of muscles and nerves. This can happen due to external compression also. This is the arteriovenous pressure gradient theory for the development of ACS [15]. A vicious cycle follows that (Appendix 1). The decreased capillary pressure leads to decreased tissue perfusion leading to increased capillary permeability and increased extravasation of fluid into the interstitial spaces further increasing the tissue pressure and decrease in tissue perfusion. A decrease in venous return also results in a decrease in tissue perfusion due to an increase in interstitial pressure [16]. When the intra-compartment pressure is more than 10 to 30 mm of Hg above the diastolic pressure tissue perfusion is compromised, and when it exceeds mean arterial pressure muscle ischemia starts. There is a direct relation between systemic blood pressure and intra-compartmental pressure in the development of ACS. Hence a hypotensive patient is more likely to develop ACS compared to normotensive [17].

Most muscle injury occurs not during the phase of ischemia but at the time of reperfusion. Ischemia–reperfusion syndrome is the cellular and systemic effects of ischemia followed by reperfusion. Normally the energy demands are met by oxidation of free fatty acids leads to aerobic conversion of ADP to ATP. During ischemia, cells try to preserve energy. Ischemia induces two anaerobic pathways for energy production. The first is from creatine phosphate stored in the muscles. The creatine kinase in the muscle produces a large amount of ATP by transferring phosphate from creatine phosphate to the ADP molecule. The creatine phosphate stores in the muscles will be depleted within three hours. The glycogen within the muscles is the next source of energy. The glycogen is broken down into pyruvate and lactate. The hydrogen ions released during this process decrease the intracellular pH. This inhibits glycolysis by negative inhibition of the rate-limiting enzyme phosphofructokinase. This is an inefficient mechanism of ATP production. This will end in six hours. Later dephosphorylation of adenosine nucleotide continues leading to the production of fat-soluble precursors like inosine monophosphate, adenosine, hypoxanthine, and xanthine. These products are washed away during reperfusion and unavailable for adenine nucleotide restoration. The vasodilation during revascularization leads to hyperemia to the extremity. This will wash away the lactate and precursors of adenine nucleotide metabolism. The hyperemia causes increased extravasation fluid through the capillaries leading to a rise in interstitial pressure. The muscles are the only tissue in which xanthene dehydrogenase is converted to xanthine oxidase during reperfusion and not during ischemia. This is due to the increased concentration of cytosolic calcium. The oxygen-free radicles produced by the xanthene oxidase react with proteins and enzymes. The free radicles attack the unsaturated bonds of free fatty acids in the phospholipid bilayer of the cell membrane called lipid peroxidation. Lipid peroxidation causes fragmentation and structural-functional alteration in the membrane leading to increased permeability. This reaction in the capillary leads to increased permeability cell swelling and interstitial edema increasing the vascular resistance. These abnormalities in the cell wall functions allow calcium influx into the cytoplasm. Increased cytoplasmic calcium will completely uncouple the oxidative phosphorylation and production of ATP in the mitochondria. This influx of calcium leads to cell death and necrosis. This reperfusion injury cascade can induce further local and systemic organ failure [18].

The irreversible changes and reduction of aerobic metabolism in the tissue due to ischemia are different for different tissues. It depends on the ischemic time which can vary from minutes to hours. Within 6 hours of acute ischemia irreversible tissue necrosis and inflammatory cascade leading to fibrosis sets in muscles. Ischemia of 1 hour produces reversible neuropraxia in nerves. Irreversible axonotmesis sets in about 4 hours of acute ischemia [19, 20].

4. Clinical features

The signs and symptoms of ACS evolve within few hours. A high index of suspicion is required for the diagnosis of ACS. Griffiths described pain, paresthesia, paresis, and pain with stretch as the main symptoms of ACS ("four Ps") later pulselessness and pink color of skin were added [21, 22]. Pain out of proportion to the known injury is the earliest symptom. Pain not responding to analgesics also make us suspicious. Resting pain and exacerbation of pain on passive stretching of affected muscles are present. Paresthesia due to ischemia of nerves can be an early sign. But an assessment of neurological functions for the diagnosis of ACS can be tricky. The extreme pain, anxiety, and altered mental status due to an injury can make proper neurological examination impossible. The motor nerve fibers can withstand the ischemia to a longer extent than sensory fibers hence motor weakness will be present at a later stage. Swelling and distension of the affected extremity should alert the surgeon about the possibility of an incumbent ACS. Resting pain or pain due to passive stretching of muscles, paresthesia, pallor, pulselessness, and paresis (5Ps) can be seen in ACS. Any one of the above signs may not be indicative of ACS. When three or more of the above signs are present in combination in a patient at risk of developing ACS will increase the sensitivity of these signs for diagnosis. Among these signs, the paresis may take longer to appear. The 5 Ps described above are characteristic features of arterial ischemia. In a conscious patient pain out of proportion to known injuries and paresthesia are the most important signs. Two-point discrimination is a more sensitive test than a light touch. Sometimes a 6th P - Poikilothermia a change in temperature of the extremity or coolness of the affected limb may be present in ACS [23]. In young children with injury, the above-mentioned features may not be useful for diagnosis. They may not be able to communicate regarding their symptoms and signs. The increasing need for analgesics, features of agitation, and anxiety (3 As) are indicators for the development of ACS. Clinical diagnosis of ACS is challenging in an unconscious patient, in a patient using patient-controlled analgesia, regional anesthesia, and use of epidural pain catheters because of masking of clinical features [24].

The leg is the most common site of acute compartment syndrome. The anterior and lateral compartments of the leg are commonly affected. Fractures of the tibia, tibial plateau fractures, and fracture-dislocations of the knee are the common injuries producing ACS of the leg. According to the compartment involved the clinical features can change. Paresthesia of the first webspace of the foot is an early sign. Later weakness of dorsiflexion of the great toe, inversion of the foot, and dorsiflexion of the ankle are seen in anterior compartment involvement. The lateral compartment syndrome produces a sensory loss in the dorsolateral aspect of the foot with weakness of eversion of the foot. Deep posterior compartment involvement leads to loss of plantar flexion of the toes with loss of sensations in the plantar aspect of the foot. Plantar flexion of the ankle will be weak when the superficial posterior compartment is affected [25].

Dislocations of Chopart and Lisfranc joints are the commonest cause for foot compartment syndrome. Isolated fractures of the mid-foot bones are a very rare cause. The symptoms are similar to leg compartment syndrome. Frequent checking of sensations especially two-point discrimination is a sensitive test. Passive stretching of muscles results in exacerbation of pain [26].

ACS of the thigh is a very rare and potentially devastating condition. Fracture of the shaft of the femur, contusion, coagulopathy, vascular injuries, intramuscular hematoma, arthroplasties of hip and knee, and arthroscopy of the knee are some of the etiologies. The outcome can be an uneventful recovery to severe morbidity and mortality. The diagnosis of ACS in a conscious patient able to cooperate with examination is based on the following criteria. Pain out of proportion to the injury, significant swelling of the thigh, palpable induration of the involved compartment, increase in measured thigh circumference, pain with passive stretching, weakness of the involved muscle, sensory or motor weakness in the nerves in the affected compartment are all seen in varying combinations in acute compartment syndrome of the thigh. An excessively painful, tensely swollen thigh is the most consistent finding of ACS of thigh [27].

The lumbar paraspinal muscle compartment syndrome can be either acute or chronic. Acute cases are due to injuries from downhill skiing, or surfing, direct injury to muscles, or lifting weight. Localized paraspinal muscle tenderness, board-like rigidity of the muscles, deep tenderness on palpation of the abdomen, absent bowel sounds, and loss of sensation over the paraspinal area are the common features. Localized loss of sensations in the paraspinal region is a pathognomonic finding [28].

Supracondylar fracture of the humerus with vascular injury is the commonest cause of ACS in the forearm. The deep volar compartment is commonly involved, flexor pollicis longus and flexor digitorum profundus are commonly involved. Trauma, crush injuries, insect bites are the commonest cause of ACS of hand. Other than the usual symptoms and signs pain on passive motion of the metacarpophalangeal joints of the corresponding intrinsic muscle is a sensitive test [29, 30].

5. Investigations

Despite the awareness among doctors about the possibility of ACS in trauma patients it is one condition frequently missed leading to devastating complications. The clinical suspicion of this condition must lead to immediate decompression without many investigations. This is especially true in an unconscious patient, intubated patients, and who cannot respond appropriately.

The compartment pressure measurement is the most common method used to diagnose ACS. The measurement of pressure should be done within 5cms from the fracture and not at the site of fracture. Compartment pressure measured over time is more useful than a single measurement. The diagnosis depends on the delta pressure measurement. Delta pressure is the difference between diastolic pressure and compartment pressure. When delta pressure is equal to or less than 30 mg of Hg it indicates ACS. If we use only delta pressure for treatment it has been shown that many asymptomatic patients will undergo fasciotomy. So diagnosis must be confirmed only with clinical findings and hemodynamic and metabolic parameters [31]. In an unconscious patient compartment pressure measurement is the only way to diagnose ACS. Compartment pressure must be checked every 4 hours in the first 24 hours in all high-risk unconscious patients after an injury.

Several techniques can be used for measuring compartment pressure. The needle manometry technique is the simplest and cheapest technique. This is introduced by whitesides et al. (1975). The Wick catheter, the slit catheter, the solid-state transducer intra- compartment catheter, myopress catheter, and transducer-tipped fiber optic catheters are other methods used [32].

The intramuscular partial pressure of oxygen can be measured noninvasively using Near-Infrared spectroscopy (NIRS). There is an increase in perfusion to the injured site. So the partial pressure of oxygen will increase at the site of injury. If there is no increase in the partial pressure of oxygen at the site of injury it can indicate ACS. This is the principle of NIRS. The intramuscular partial pressure of oxygen can vary among individuals and different compartments. A comparison of the NIRS value of the same compartment of the opposite uninjured leg is a useful tool for diagnosis. There is some controversy regarding the use of NIRS for the monitoring of ACS. Different factors like depth of tissues, discoloration of the skin, a hematoma can interfere with the results of NIRS [33].

Many different techniques are used for detecting compartment pressure and perfusion but they are still in the development or experimental stage. Ultrasonography can show increased echogenicity of the compartment when pressure increases. It can also be used to detect changes in elasticity when standardized external pressure is applied. Both techniques are in an experimental stage. Pulse Phased Locked Loop (PPLL) ultrasound is useful in detecting the displacement of fascia with arterial pulsation. This technique was found to be useful to detect raised compartment pressure in cadaveric studies. Photoplethysmography, laser Doppler flowmetry, and scintigraphy, intramuscular glucose monitoring are all used to find out raised compartment pressure. They are not used widely in clinical practice [34].

The serum biomarkers are used for the diagnosis of ACS without many shreds of evidence. Elevated Troponin Levels and myoglobinuria can assist in the diagnosis of ACS. There are also reports suggesting the usefulness of lactate levels from femoral veins in the diagnosis of ACS in patients with femoral artery injury. Serum biomarkers are not useful in the delayed diagnosis of ACS [35]. The creatine kinase level increases during ACS. Creatine kinase level > 1000 U/ml or myoglobinuria are suggestive of ACS. There are abnormalities in renal function tests and hyperkalemia due to rhabdomyolysis [36].

6. Treatment

Acute compartment syndrome is a surgical emergency. If not diagnosed early and treated promptly it can lead to devastating complications. The sequel of untreated or mismanaged ACS includes unacceptable deformities, neurological injuries, crush syndrome, renal failure, limb amputation, and death. There are certain preventive measures that we should do to prevent the development of acute compartment syndrome in all patients with limb injuries. All circumferential and tight bandages should be removed. Split tight plaster cast. The Limb should be kept at heart level. Avoid patient going into hypotension, and maintain oxygen saturation. These measures reduce the risk of the development of ACS in high-risk patients.

The treatment of ACS is emergency decompression of the compartment. The fasciotomy is used for decompression. Fasciotomy should be done within 6 hours or definitely within 12 hours after diagnosis of ACS. Fasciotomy must be done in all patients with clinical findings of ACS when compartment pressure is more than 30 mm of Hg, and when delta pressure is less than or equal to 30 mm of Hg. The fasciotomy should be liberal decompressing all the compartments of the limb including the epimysium to relieve integumental compartment pressure. In the legs all 4 compartments, and the forearm, both dorsal and volar compartments should be decompressed. The fasciotomy wound can be closed by delayed primary intension, or by a split-thickness skin graft. The use of negative pressure wound therapy for fasciotomy wounds is controversial. It can help to reduce the swelling and early closure of wounds or skin grafting. A fasciotomy is not indicated when there is irreversible intra-compartmental damage like neuromuscular or vascular damage in an adult patient. If fracture fixation is needed in such a patient either external fixation or plaster cast can be used without violating the affected compartment. In a patient with ACS fracture fixation, either internal or external fixation can be done along with fasciotomy [35, 37]. In children, delayed fasciotomies have shown better outcomes than adults. We can do fasciotomies up to 24 hours after injury in children [38].

ACS of the leg is common in the fractures of the diaphysis, proximal fracture of tibia with comminution, long periarticular fragments, fracture-dislocations, and medial tibial condyle fractures. Comminuted fracture of the fibula at the same level of fracture of tibia is also associated with a high incidence of ACS [39].

All four compartments have to be decompressed. The commonly used 2 incision technique involves a longitudinal incision on the posteromedial aspect of the leg extending from the proximal tibia to distally up to the musculotendinous junction of the gastro-soleus muscle. The incision is made 2 cm posterior to the postero-medial corner of the tibia. Care should be taken to avoid injuring the sural nerve proximally and saphenous vein distally. The fascia is incised in line with incision decompressing the superficial compartment. The deep compartment is decompressed by elevating the soleus muscle and cutting the fascia covering it. We can extend the incision proximally and distally as needed for the release. The second incision is made 2 cm anterior to the head of the fibula. The incision extends from the head of the fibula to the distal fibula. The anterior skin flap is raised and the lateral intermuscular septum is identified and the anterior compartment is released by incising the entire length of the facia from proximal to distal. The superficial peroneal nerve is at risk at the distal third. The lateral compartment is released by incising the fascia along the posterior border of the fibula (**Figure 1**) [40].

A single incision technique can be used for the fasciotomy of the leg. A longitudinal incision is made along the entire length of the fibula. A transverse incision is made to identify the lateral intermuscular septum then decompression of the anterior and lateral compartment is done. The posterior compartment is decompressed after elevating the attachment of the soleus from the fibula and then identifing the posterior compartment and decompressing it. Fibulectomy can be used to decompress all 4 compartments of the leg, but it should be avoided especially in patients with complex tibial fractures [41].

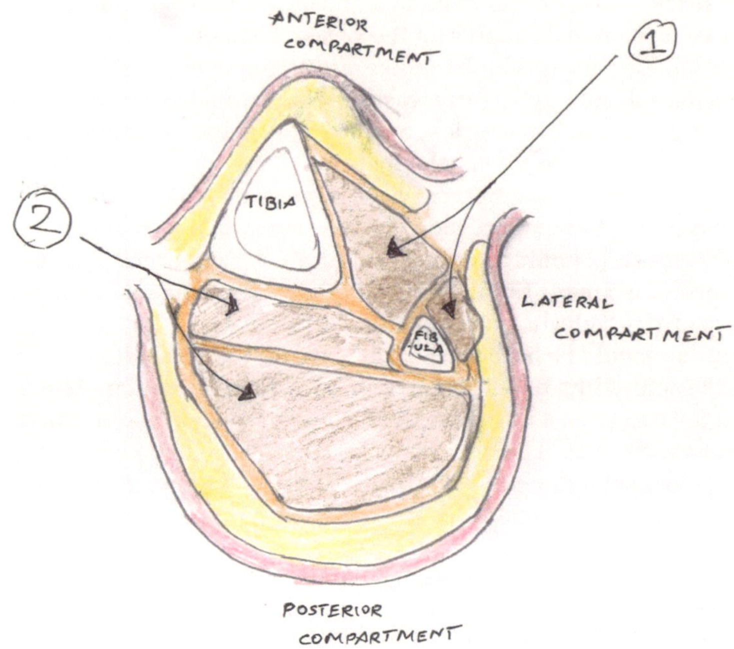

Figure 1.
Diagram showing the compartments of the leg and arrows 1 & 2 represent the approach for the fasciotomy of the leg.

There are different methods for fasciotomy of the foot. The most commonly used method is a combination of medial and dorsal approaches. The dorsal approach involves two longitudinal incisions one medial to the second metatarsal and another lateral to the fourth metatarsal. There should be adequate space between these 2 incisions to prevent necrosis of the skin. The medial incision is about 6 cm long starting from about 4 cm anterior to heel and about 3 cm above the plantar surface of the foot. The dorsal approach helps to decompress the interossei and adductor compartments (**Figure 2**). The medial approach releases the medial, superficial, calcaneal, and lateral compartments [42].

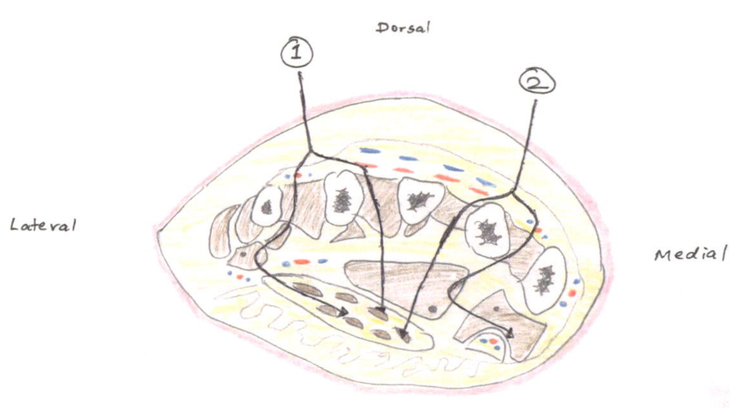

Figure 2.
Dorsal approach for fasciotomy of the foot- a cross-section.

The decompression of all three compartments is indicated in ACS of the thigh. The anterior and posterior compartments are decompressed using a single lateral incision extending from the intertrochanteric line to the lateral epicondyle of the femur. The skin and subcutaneous tissue are opened along the skin incision. The iliotibial band is identified. By dividing the iliotibial band fascia covering the vastus lateralis the anterior compartment is released. The posterior compartment is opened after retracting the vastus lateralis and dividing the intermuscular septum. The medial compartment is decompressed using a separate longitudinal medial incision and dividing the medial intermuscular septum (**Figure 3**) [43].

The paraspinal muscles are enclosed in the thoracolumbar fascia which acts as a closed fascial compartment. It covers the muscles from all sides except medially where it is attached to the spinous process and interspinous ligaments (**Figure 4**). Surgical release of the thoracolumbar fascia gives better results than nonoperative treatment in the compartment syndrome of the paraspinal muscles. There is no consensus regarding the timing of fasciotomy. Most reports agree on fasciotomy within 7 days. The approach is Wiltse paraspinal incision. The thoracolumbar fascia is divided and individual muscle compartments are released [44].

The management of ACS of the forearm involves decompression of the compartment using volar and dorsal approaches. The volar incision is curvilinear. It extends from proximal and medal to cubital fossa then extends distally along the radial side of the forearm till the distal third. Then again it is curved medially to the midline of the forearm over the wrist for release of carpal tunnel (**Figure 5**). This incision helps to decompress the median nerve and helps to cover the median nerve using the radial flap. The lacertus fibrous is released and the superficial volar compartment is released. The identification of the deep fascia and its release is very important. The pronator quadratus should be identified and its fascia should be released separately. The dorsal compartment is decompressed using a single midline incision

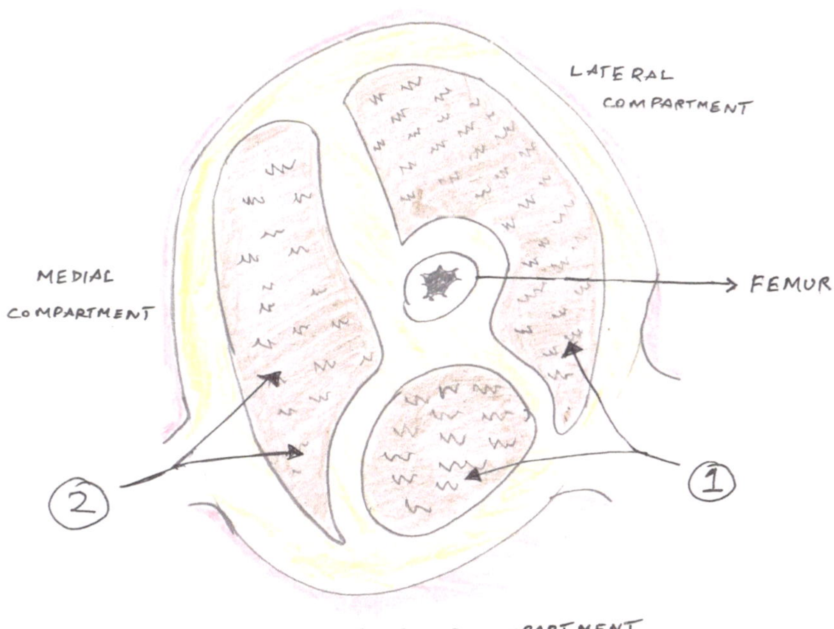

Figure 3.
The anterior, lateral, and posterior compartments of the thigh and arrows representing the lateral and medial fasciotomy approaches.

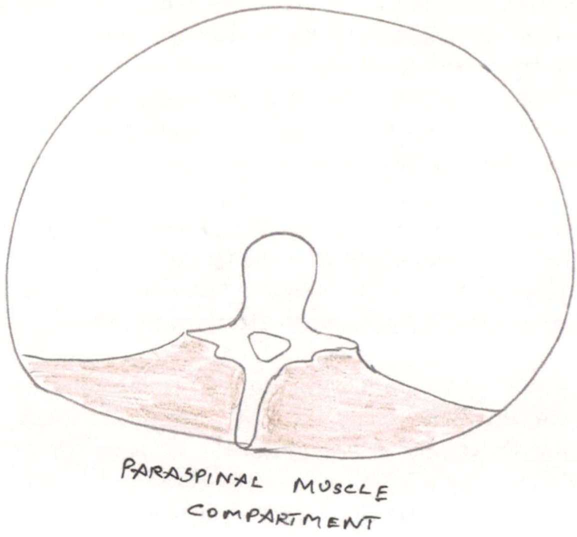

Figure 4.
Diagram showing the paraspinal muscle compartment, the thoracodorsal fascia covering the muscles all around and medially to the spinous process and interspinous ligaments.

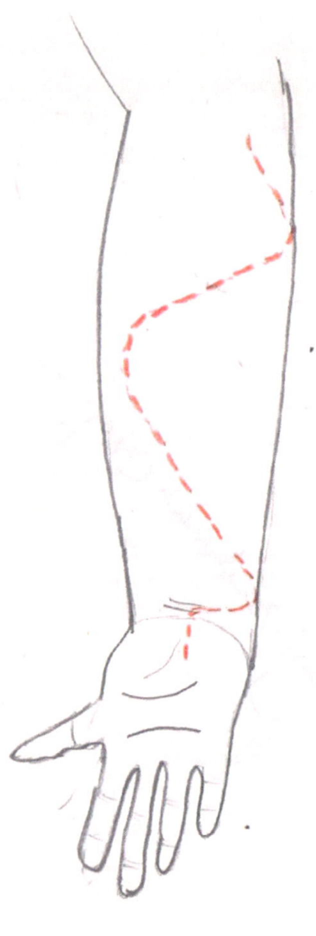

Figure 5.
The volar approach for fasciotomy of the forearm.

extending from lateral epicondyle to distal radioulnar joint. The individual septum separating the muscles should be released individually [45].

The hand compartment is released by the volar and dorsal approach. Dorsally decompression is done using 2 incisions along the 2nd and 4th metacarpals. The release is done on either side of the metacarpals to decompress the interossei. Deeper dissection along the radial aspect of the 2nd metacarpal is used for decompressing the adductor compartment. The volar incision is used to release the thenar and hypothenar compartments. The carpal tunnel should also be released [46].

7. Conclusion

Acute compartment syndrome is a surgical emergency. The diagnosis is based on clinical findings so careful history and physical examination are required. In obtunded patients, the diagnosis is made when delta pressure ≤ 30mm of Hg and compartment pressure > 30 mm of Hg. Emergency fasciotomy and decompression of the compartment is the treatment of choice. Usually, a repeat inspection of the fasciotomy wound after 24 to 48 hours should be done. Delayed closure of the wound is done.

Appendix 1: The vicious cycle in the pathogenesis of acute compartment syndrome

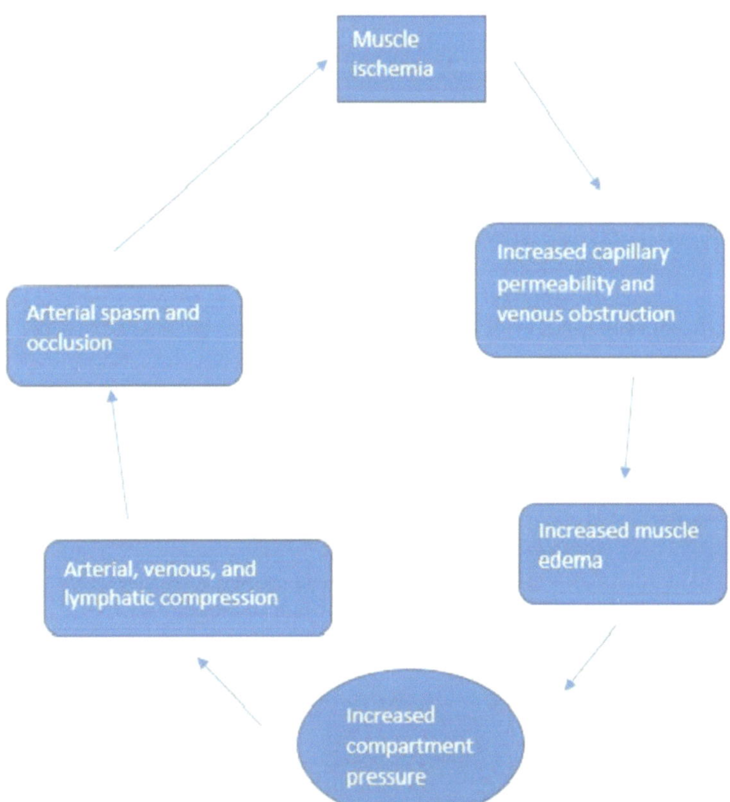

Author details

Balaji Zacharia* and Raj Vignesh Selvaraj
Department of Orthopedics, Government Medical College,
Kozhikode, Kerala, India

*Address all correspondence to: balaji.zacharia@gmail.com

References

[1] Garner MR, Taylor SA, GausdTen E, Lyden JP. Compartment syndrome: diagnosis, management, and unique concerns in the twenty-first century. HSS J. 2014;10(2):143-152. doi:10.1007/s11420-014-9386-8

[2] R. Volkmann, "Die ischaemischen Muskellähmungen und Kontrakturen," Zentralblatt für Chirurgie, vol. 8, pp. 801-803, 1881.

[3] McQueen MM, Gaston P, Court-Brown CM. Acute compartment syndrome. The Journal of Bone and Joint Surgery British volume. 2000;82-B(2):200-203. doi:10.1302/0301-620x.82b2.0820200

[4] Stahel PF, Mauser N, Gissel H, Henderson C, Hao J, Mauffrey C. Acute Lower-leg Compartment Syndrome. Orthopedics. 2013;36(8):619-624. doi:10.3928/01477447-20130724-07

[5] Taylor RM, Sullivan MP, Mehta S. Acute compartment syndrome: obtaining diagnosis, providing treatment, and minimizing medicolegal risk. Curr Rev Musculoskelet Med. 2012;5(3):206-213. doi:10.1007/s12178-012-9126-y

[6] Stella M, Santolini E, Sanguineti F, et al. Aetiology of trauma-related acute compartment syndrome of the leg: A systematic review. Injury. 2019;50:S57-S64. doi:10.1016/j.injury.2019.01.047

[7] Hutchinson, M.R., Ireland, M.L. Common Compartment Syndromes in Athletes. Sports Med. 17, 200-208 (1994). https://doi.org/10.2165/00007256-199417030-00006

[8] Hope MJ, McQueen MM. Acute compartment syndrome in the absence of fracture. J Orthop Trauma. 2004 Apr;18(4):220-4. doi: 10.1097/00005131-200404000-00005. PMID: 15087965.

[9] Hasnain Raza, Anant Mahapatra, "Acute Compartment Syndrome in Orthopedics: Causes, Diagnosis, and Management", Advances in Orthopedics, vol. 2015, Article ID 543412, 8 pages, 2015. https://doi.org/10.1155/2015/543412

[10] Pechar J, Lyons MM. Acute Compartment Syndrome of the Lower Leg: A Review. The Journal for Nurse Practitioners. 2016;12(4):265-270. doi:10.1016/j.nurpra.2015.10.013

[11] Frink, M., Hildebrand, F., Krettek, C. et al. Compartment Syndrome of the Lower Leg and Foot. Clin Orthop Relat Res , 940-950 (2010). https://doi.org/10.1007/s11999-009-0891-x

[12] Ronel, Daniel N. M.D.; Mtui, Estomih M.D.; Nolan, William B. III M.D. Forearm Compartment Syndrome: Anatomical Analysis of Surgical Approaches to the Deep Space, Plastic and Reconstructive Surgery: September 1, 2004 - Volume 114 - Issue 3 - p 697-705 doi: 10.1097/01.PRS.0000130967.42426.23

[13] Ling, Marcus Z. X. M.B.B.S.; Kumar, V P. F.R.C.S. Myofascial Compartments of the Hand in Relation to Compartment Syndrome: A Cadaveric Study, Plastic and Reconstructive Surgery: February 2009 - Volume 123 - Issue 2 - p 613-616 doi: 10.1097/PRS.0b013e3181956538

[14] Nadeem RD, Clift BA, Martindale JP, Hadden WA, Ritchie IK. Acute compartment syndrome of the thigh after joint replacement with anticoagulation. The Journal of Bone and Joint Surgery British volume. 1998;80-B(5):866-868. doi:10.1302/0301-620x.80b5.0800866

[15] Elliott KGB, Johnstone AJ. DIAGNOSING ACUTE COMPARTMENT SYNDROME. The Journal of Bone and Joint Surgery British volume. 2003;85-B(5):625-632. doi:10.1302/0301-620x.85b5.14352

[16] Oak NR, Abrams RA. Compartment Syndrome of the Hand. Orthopedic

Clinics of North America. 2016;47(3): 609-616. doi:10.1016/j.ocl.2016.03.006

[17] Olson SA, Glasgow RR. Acute Compartment Syndrome in Lower Extremity Musculoskeletal Trauma. Journal of the American Academy of Orthopaedic Surgeons. 2005;13(7):436-444. doi:10.5435/00124635-200511000-00003

[18] T. Tollens, H. Janzing & P. Broos (1998) The Pathophysiology of the Acute Compartment Syndrome, Acta Chirurgica Belgica, 98:4, 171-175, DOI: 10.1080/00015458.1998.12098409

[19] Hargens AR, Romine JS, Sipe JC, Evans KL, Mubarak SJ, Akeson WH. Peripheral nerve-conduction block by high muscle-compartment pressure. The Journal of Bone & Joint Surgery. 1979;61(2):192-200. doi:10.2106/00004623-197961020-00006

[20] HUARD J, LI Y, FU FH. MUSCLE INJURIES AND REPAIR. The Journal of Bone and Joint Surgery-American Volume. 2002;84(5):822-832. doi:10.2106/00004623-200205000-00022

[21] Griffiths DLl. THE MANAGEMENT OF ACUTE CIRCULATORY FAILURE IN AN INJURED LIMB. The Journal of Bone and Joint Surgery British volume. 1948;30-B(2):280-289. doi:10.1302/0301-620x.30b2.280

[22] Cascio BM, Wilckens JH, Ain MC, Toulson C, Frassica FJ. Documentation of Acute Compartment Syndrome at an Academic Health-Care Center. The Journal of Bone & Joint Surgery. 2005; 87(2):346-350. doi:10.2106/jbjs.d.02007

[23] Murdock M, Murdoch MM. Compartment Syndrome: A Review of the Literature. Clinics in Podiatric Medicine and Surgery. 2012;29(2):301-310. doi:10.1016/j.cpm.2012.02.001

[24] von Keudell AG, Weaver MJ, Appleton PT, et al. Diagnosis and treatment of acute extremity compartment syndrome. The Lancet. 2015;386(10000):1299-1310. doi: 10.1016/s0140-6736(15)00277-9

[25] Pechar J, Lyons MM. Acute Compartment Syndrome of the Lower Leg: A Review. J Nurse Pract. 2016; 12(4):265-270. doi:10.1016/j.nurpra.2015.10.013

[26] Frink M, Hildebrand F, Krettek C, Brand J, Hankemeier S. Compartment syndrome of the lower leg and foot. Clin Orthop Relat Res. 2010;468(4):940-950. doi:10.1007/s11999-009-0891-x

[27] Mith??fer K, Lhowe DW, Vrahas MS, Altman DT, Altman GT. Clinical Spectrum of Acute Compartment Syndrome of the Thigh and Its Relation to Associated Injuries. Clinical Orthopaedics and Related Research. 2004;425:223-229. doi:10.1097/00003086-200408000-00032

[28] Nathan ST, Roberts CS, Deliberato D. Lumbar paraspinal compartment syndrome. International Orthopaedics (SICOT). 2012;36(6):1221-1227. doi:10.1007/s00264-011-1386-4

[29] Botte MJ, Gelberman RH. ACUTE COMPARTMENT SYNDROME OF THE FOREARM. Hand Clinics. 1998;14(3): 391-403. doi:10.1016/s0749-0712(21)00398-x

[30] Codding JL, Vosbikian MM, Ilyas AM. Acute Compartment Syndrome of the Hand. The Journal of Hand Surgery. 2015;40(6):1213-1216. doi:10.1016/j.jhsa.2015.01.034

[31] McMillan TE, Gardner WT, Schmidt AH, Johnstone AJ. Diagnosing acute compartment syndrome—where have we got to? International Orthopaedics (SICOT). 2019;43(11):2429-2435. doi:10.1007/s00264-019-04386-y

[32] Beniwal RK, Bansal A. Osteofascial compartment pressure measurement in

closed limb injuries – Whitesides' technique revisited. Journal of Clinical Orthopaedics and Trauma. 2016;7(4):225-228. doi:10.1016/j.jcot.2016.01.001

[33] Bariteau JT, Beutel BG, Kamal R, Hayda R, Born C. The Use of Near-Infrared Spectrometry for the Diagnosis of Lower-extremity Compartment Syndrome. Orthopedics. 2011;34(3):178-178. doi:10.3928/01477447-20110124-12

[34] McMillan TE, Gardner WT, Schmidt AH, Johnstone AJ. Diagnosing acute compartment syndrome—where have we got to? International Orthopaedics (SICOT). 2019;43(11):2429-2435. doi:10.1007/s00264-019-04386-y

[35] Osborn, Col. Patrick M. MD; Schmidt, Andrew H. MD Management of Acute Compartment Syndrome, Journal of the American Academy of Orthopaedic Surgeons: February 1, 2020 - Volume 28 - Issue 3 - p e108-e114 doi: 10.5435/JAAOS-D-19-00270

[36] Long B, Koyfman A, Gottlieb M. Evaluation and Management of Acute Compartment Syndrome in the Emergency Department. The Journal of Emergency Medicine. 2019;56(4):386-397. doi:10.1016/j.jemermed.2018.12.021

[37] Wall CJ, Lynch J, Harris IA, et al. Clinical practice guidelines for the management of acute limb compartment syndrome following trauma. 2010; 80(3):151-156. doi:10.1111/j.1445-2197.2010.05213.x

[38] Lin JS, Samora JB. Pediatric acute compartment syndrome: a systematic review and meta-analysis. 2020;29(1):90-96. doi:10.1097/bpb.0000000000000593

[39] Stella M, Santolini E, Sanguineti F, et al. Aetiology of trauma-related acute compartment syndrome of the leg: A systematic review. Injury. 2019;50:S57-S64. doi:10.1016/j.injury.2019.01.047

[40] Konda SR, Kester BS, Fisher N, Behery OA, Crespo AM, Egol KA. Acute Compartment Syndrome of the Leg. 2017;31(3):S17-S18. doi:10.1097/bot.0000000000000894

[41] Köstler W, Strohm PC, Südkamp NP. Acute compartment syndrome of the limb. Injury. 2005;36(8):992-998. doi:10.1016/j.injury.2005.01.007

[42] Fulkerson E, Razi A, Tejwani N. Review: Acute Compartment Syndrome of the Foot. Foot Ankle Int. 2003;24(2):180-187. doi:10.1177/107110070302400214

[43] Ojike NI, Roberts CS, Giannoudis PV. Compartment syndrome of the thigh: A systematic review. Injury. 2010;41(2):133-136. doi:10.1016/j.injury.2009.03.016

[44] Alexander W, Low N, Pratt G. Acute lumbar paraspinal compartment syndrome: a systematic review. ANZ J Surg. 2018;88(9):854-859. doi:10.1111/ans.14342

[45] Kistler JM, Ilyas AM, Thoder JJ. Forearm Compartment Syndrome. Hand Clinics. 2018;34(1):53-60. doi:10.1016/j.hcl.2017.09.006

[46] Rubinstein AJ, Ahmed IH, Vosbikian MM. Hand Compartment Syndrome. Hand Clinics. 2018;34(1):41-52. doi:10.1016/j.hcl.2017.09.005

Section 6

Burn and COVID-19

Chapter 8

Management and Clinical Aspects of Burned Patients Affected by SARS-COV2

Filippo Andrea Giovanni Perozzo, Alex Pontini, Alberto De Lazzari, Alvise Montanari, Giovanni Valotto and Bruno Azzena

Abstract

At the end of January 2020, SARS-CoV-2 started escalating worldwide. COVID-19 can exert its effects on immunity, inflammation, and multi-organ system disease, common denominators with the burn injury. The pandemic required major efforts to Burn centres in order to preserve burn patients' care and contribute to the health care response. In our Burn Unit we autonomously developed a protocol for patients acceptance and surveillance of the hospitalized ones and the personnel. We briefly describe our experience with six cases of burn patients infected by SARS-CoV-2 highlighting the overlap between medical treatment of burn patients and COVID-19 patients. To avoid viral spreading epidemiologic control is essential, especially preventive measures such as isolation of infected patients and identification of the source of infection. In our surgical practice, we increased the use of enzymatic debridement avoiding procedures with a high risk of viral particles spreading. Personnel protection and dedicated pathways have been planned, optimizing air circulation and disinfection. Vaccines represent the best hope for the global population to stop the viral spread, despite new variants outbreaks.

Keywords: COVID-19, Burn Unit, Burn Patients, Preventive measures, Clinical and surgical management, experience

1. Introduction

1.1 Background

At the beginning of December 2019 was reported for the first time, in the city of Wuhan, Central China, a pneumonia of unknown origin, named "coronavirus disease 2019" (COVID-19), caused by an agent initially known as 2019 novel coronavirus (2019-nCOV) and later referred as severe acute respiratory syndrome coronavirus 2 (SARS-CoV-2) [1].

1.2 Epidemiology

Since the end of January 2020, SARS-CoV-2 started escalating worldwide until it was declared a pandemic disease by the World Health Organization on

March 11th, 2020. By the end of May 2020, the disease reached 188 countries causing nearly 370000 deaths. In Italy, clusters of cases were detected on 21th and 22th of February 2020 only in the regions of Lombardy and Veneto. At the beginning of March 2020, the virus was present in all regions of Italy leading the government to quarantine the whole population. For more than a year, Italy has been burdened by a huge number of cases and deaths with a related increase in hospitalizations and ICU admissions leading to a consequent constant hard stress for the National Health System. Meanwhile, scientists from all over the world intensively strived to unravel virus characteristics and develop new therapeutic and preventive approaches.

1.3 SARS-CoV-2 and burned patients

Since the COVID-19 epidemic onset, SARS-CoV-2 demonstrated a major contagious capability [2] with recent findings demonstrating possible similar pathophysiological features with SARS-CoV [3].

The mechanism of infection among humans is based on inhaled respiratory droplets with the virus replicating in the nasopharyngeal mucosa, spreading then into the lungs with lower respiratory tract infection capability. Close contact could also represent an infection source through mucosal surfaces of the nose, mouth, and eyes [4, 5]. Besides, there is also the chance of aerosol transmission in a closed environment.

Viremia, after the entrance of the virus in the circulatory system, can provoke secondary involvement of various target organs (e.g., heart, kidney, and central nervous system) with pathophysiological effects of SARS-CoV-2 ranging from acute lung injury to systemic and pulmonary hypertension, heightened inflammation, vascular hyperpermeability, coagulopathy and cardiovascular and gastrointestinal complications [3, 6].

Among the various types of trauma, extended burns can be considered as one of the most dramatic ones, characterized by a state of hypermetabolism with a catabolic shift, a state of hyperdynamic circulation and inflammation, subsequently linked to multiorgan failure and poor outcome [7, 8]. Additional pathophysiologic changes include vascular leaking mediated by polymorphonuclear activation and hemodynamic instability [9]. Moreover, immunosuppression, reported in major burn injuries [10], can determine a higher risk of infections which in turn can degenerate into sepsis, multiorgan failure and death.

Patient's age, total body surface area with burns, inhalation injury, and arising organ dysfunction are some of the principal prognosis predictors of burns [4, 11, 12].

In this way, COVID-19 can exert its effects on immunity, inflammation, and multi-organ system disease, common denominators with the burn injury, especially because SARS-CoV-2 infection might be a concurrent disease in a patient presenting to the medical attention for burns, needing immediate evaluation and medical attention even before COVID- 19 can be ruled out.

2. Burn unit experience during the pandemic period

COVID-19 disease, when symptomatic, usually presents itself with fever, cough, and myalgia or fatigue. Less common presentations are sputum production, sore throat, nasal congestion, anosmia, headache, hemoptysis, and diarrhea [13]. The severe pattern of evolution is characterized by worsening dyspnoea with hypoxemia and lymphopenia after which septic shock, ARDS, metabolic acidosis, and coagulation dysfunction can rapidly develop [14].

The actual pandemic pushed Burn centres efforts forward, keeping a fair balance between preserving burn patients' care and contributing to the health care response.

Due to the lack of really effective therapies and prevention measures such as vaccination during the virus initial outbreak, the major and most effective ways for disease spreading control were the isolation of affected patients, tracing of infected, hands hygiene, respiratory airways protection, and surface sterilization [15].

Our Burn Center, located in the North-East of Italy, a third level facility responsible for the acceptance and treatment of all major burns in an area with a population of approximately 5 million people, consists of three separate units: an ICU, a semi-ICU, and a Burn and Plastic Surgery Ward. There is also an outpatient clinic for post-discharge follow-up and small interventional procedures.

Due to the high demand of personnel and resources in the semi-ICUs and ICUs, all non-emergent activity was reduced in order to allocate the resources needed. In Plastic Surgery, only major oncological and trauma cases were scheduled [16]. Our Burn Unit reduced its elective activity of correction of burn sequelae. However, urgent and emergent activities greatly increased at the beginning of the pandemic since burn patients could not be accepted by all other centres in Italy.

The incessant incoming of patients from different locations within the pandemic epicenter represented an increased risk both for patients in the Burn Unit and for healthcare workers, due to COVID19 rapid spreading inside and outside the University Hospital.

In order to face the risk of viral spread, since the beginning of the emergency period, we autonomously developed in our Burn Unit a protocol for the acceptance of all the new patients and the surveillance of the hospitalized ones and the personnel, with distinctions made for the pediatric population [17]. These measures were later followed by the general prevention and management indications established by the Medical Direction of our University Hospital. Both these protocols were in accordance and regularly updated with the most recent Italian Government and International literature guidelines [18, 19].

2.1 Burn unit admission management and COVID-19 protocol

The burn-injured patient is firstly transferred from the place of injury to the closest hospital with an emergency facility. Here, the first treatment is provided to the patient. Meanwhile, our Unit is activated and we give our first telephone consultation, predisposing the transfer to our facility if deemed necessary.

During the pandemic, non-essential visits to inpatients were suspended. To partially compensate for the loss of direct contact, we provided our patients with the possibility of phone or video calls, improving the communication of the medical personnel with their relatives about clinical conditions and future therapeutic programs.

Cornerstones of our admission protocol are the use of PPE, patients' history, rapid disease screening and identification in a dedicated room until the test response and further patient isolation with frequent reevaluations during the following 14 days after admission in the BU.

Patient admission in our centre is performed exclusively in the operating room, using PPE when necessary [20]. All patients referred to our Burn Unit, before admission to the Ward, semi-ICU and ICU, must be tested through RT-PCR nasopharyngeal swab in the sending hospital when the response timing does not interfere with patient's care or in our hospital.

Immediately after collection, samples are sent for examination at the Microbiology lab and the results are available in about 90 minutes.

In addition, only for pediatric cases, also the caregiver is tested: outside the operating room if the arrival of the patient and the caregiver is simultaneous, in the monitoring room if it is delayed.

A history of fever, cough, other COVID-19 presentation symptoms [13] or contact with suspected or confirmed COVID-19 cases, are the first indicators of the necessity of isolation of a patient even if the test performed is negative.

During the wait for the result, the patient is treated as a suspect case, in a dedicated room or in the operating room, if intubated.

Chest X-ray and routine panel of blood tests including C-Reactive Protein are performed in patients requiring admission, regardless of symptoms.

Moreover, hospital personnel employs all the appropriate protections according to the specific-setting contagion risk [21, 22], which, in particular, is higher during aerosol-generating procedures as collection of diagnostic respiratory specimens for COVID-19, intubation, extubation, manual ventilation, suctioning of the respiratory tract, tracheostomy, bronchoscopy and surgery [23, 24].

In the case of a ventilated patient, we also perform a BAL which can allow the detection of a positive case even with a negative swab result. At the end of the admission procedure, the patient is managed according to the test result (**Table 1**). If the patient is intubated, during the test waiting period he is not moved from the operating room with any more emergencies treated in the same operating block in order to avoid contamination risk to other health workers and patients.

In some cases, when the number of required tests inside the Hospital is substantial, particularly in the period of acute emergency when the waiting time for the result was prolonged, the non-intubated patient could be temporarily moved to a dedicated and isolated room equipped as a Burn Unit room.

In the case of a pediatric positive patient and a negative caregiver, only the patient is hospitalized in a "COVID-19 room", a room designed for positive patients outside Burn Unit, supplied with the same equipment as the Burn Unit rooms and assistance guaranteed by Burn Unit personnel.

Instead, if the pediatric patient is negative and the caregiver positive, the patient is hospitalized in the monitoring room for up to 48 h and a new caregiver is designated. The former caregiver is invited to return home and adopt isolation measures keeping in contact with the local authorities. The Burn Unit physician has to inform the Epidemiology service of the caregiver positivity. The new caregiver and the patient have to be tested with the nasopharyngeal swab and if the result is negative they are both admitted outside the Burn Unit and placed in the isolation room for 14 days.

If the pediatric patient is intubated, no caregiver is included as in ICUs access is denied to anyone who does not belong to healthcare personnel.

Confirmed SARS-Cov-2 affected patients are admitted to the COVID-19 Unit, in separate airborne infection isolation rooms. Critical Burn patients are placed in the COVID-19 ICU.

Infectious disease specialists are consulted early with constant participation in patient care.

Burn patients who develop symptoms after admission are isolated and undergo swab PCR analysis and chest X-ray. Isolation is maintained until definitive results are received.

Negative patients are finally moved to the Burn Unit and quarantined for the following 14 days in a single-bed room. During this period, they are tested daily for fever and COVID-19-like symptoms. These measures are also effective for the caregiver of the pediatric patient. Moreover, a second nasopharyngeal swab is performed after 48 h in suspect cases and every 7 days after admittance, according to the fact that incubation period of SARS-CoV-2 is estimated to be 3–7 days

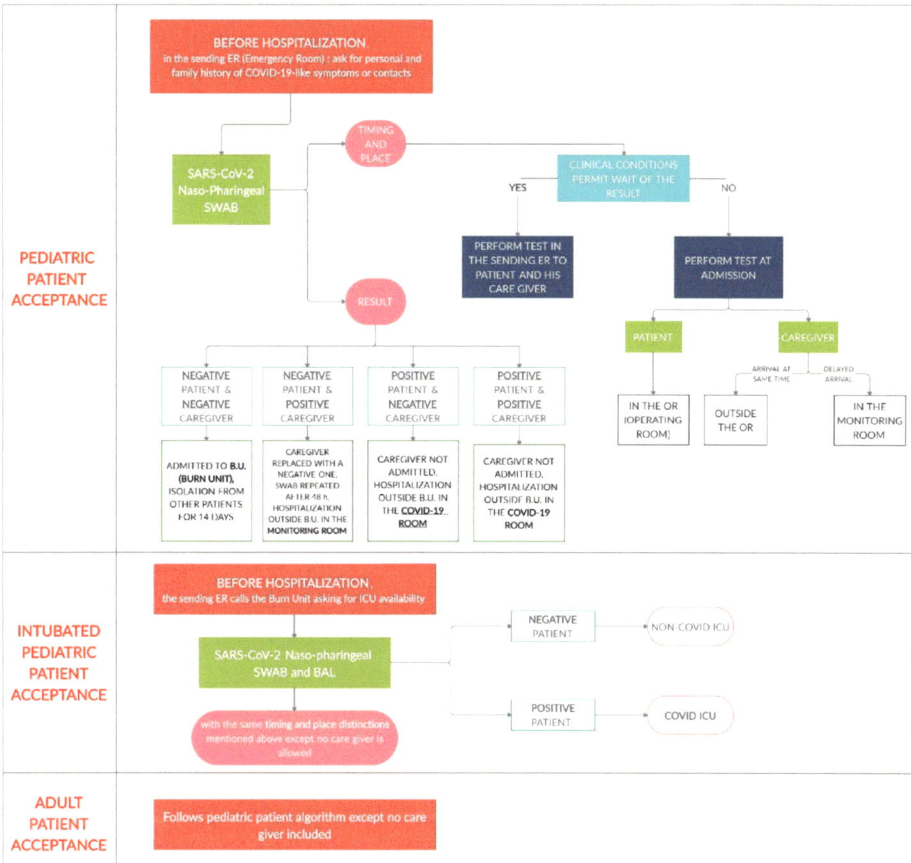

Table 1.
Acceptance protocol for pediatric and adult patients admitted to Padua university hospital burn unit.

with a range period from 2 to 14 days [25]. Both patients and caregivers are not permitted to leave the Burn Unit.

The temperature of all staff is measured at the entrance and exit from the Unit.

Unnecessary meetings are avoided with the preference given to the video conference modality.

On discharge, telemedicine follow-up is emphasized with special attention to rehabilitation.

After the initial viral pandemic spreading, in which all elective activity was suspended, we progressively began to reschedule this activity since May 2020. In order to achieve it, we have decided to screen patients first by phone and again immediately before the hospital admittance for travel history, presence of affected family members, evidence of fever or any respiratory tract symptoms in the previous weeks. In addition, asymptomatic patients undergo RT-PCR Sars-CoV-2 test before hospital admission.

2.2 Burn unit COVID-19 case series

Since the pandemic began, the main goal of our protocol was to preserve burn patients from infection and to avoid viral spread in such a delicate unit.

In the last year, from the beginning of the pandemic, 93 patients were hospitalized in our Burn Unit, including six cases of burn patients affected by SARS-CoV-2:

three of them were hospitalized with a molecular swab positive for COVID-19, while three of them were infected during the hospitalization (**Table 2**).

In April 2020 an extensive burned patient was the first to test positive for COVID-19.

She was a 56-year-old female who got burned after a domestic accident (explosion of a gas cylinder) on April 5th 2020 with 70% of TBSA. She was immediately intubated, a urinary catheter was introduced, a central line was put and fluid resuscitation was immediately commenced.

She reported a 70% TBSA burn involving face (II degree burn), neck, trunk, and upper and lower limbs (III degree burns). Once she arrived in our operating room, she immediately underwent surgical debridement of all third-degree burns and xifo–pubic and both upper limbs fasciotomies were performed. She also underwent enzymatic debridement (Nexobrid®) on her third-degree burns on the neck, shoulders, and abdomen.

A molecular swab and a BAL were performed at the arrival in the operating room and the patient stayed there until the result showed positivity for SARS-CoV-2. Finally, the patient was transferred to our COVID-19 ICU. Before the burn accident, the patient had only a mild fever (38°C), with no other symptoms reported. She got infected by her sister with whom she lived.

Once she arrived in our COVID-19 ICU her vital parameters were stabilized and she immediately underwent specific treatment for burn patient: intravenous fluid resuscitation with Ringer lactate's solution according to Parkland formula, empiric intravenous antibiotics, Low Molecular Weight Heparin (LMWH) 4000 UI once a

Age	Sex	TBSA	Covid test at hospitalization	ICU	Surgical treatment	Days of hospitalization	Positivity	Outcome
56	F	70%	+	YES	Proteolytic debridement, surgical debridement, tracheostomy, skin graftings	105	12 days	death
73	M	60%	+	YES	Proteolytic debridement, surgical debridement, skin graftings	105	3 days	death
54	M	25%	—	YES	Arm amputation, surgical debridement, skin graftings	144	52 days	healed
61	M	51%	—	YES	Surgical debridement, skin graftings	170	52 days	healed
51	F	10%	+	NO	Grafing with amniotic membrane	6	6 days	healed
25	F	41%	+	YES	Surgical debridement, skin graftings	96	5 days	healed

Table 2.
Features of our Covid-positive patients.

day, analgesic therapy and human endovenous Immunoglobulin (Pentaglobin®). In order to stabilize the vital parameters, it was necessary to perform blood and plasma transfusions and to administer noradrenaline. She was also set on an air fluidized bed (Clinitron®) for extensive burns of her back.

Initial assessment included a routine blood test, Arterial Blood Gas (ABG) every two hours, chest x-ray twice a day and rectal swab searching for MDROs.

Blood tests showed mild leukocytosis (12,02 10^9/L), implementation of PCT (0,65 ug/L), important augmentation of myolysis markers (P-CPK 5.813 U/L, P-myoglobin 3.814 ug/L).

Because of the important muscular necrosis, she rapidly developed acute kidney insufficiency and needed immediate CVVH-DF substitutive renal therapy.

Even though she initially had no Covid-like symptoms but fever, her chest x-ray showed an interstitial involvement, her lungs were less expanded and her costophrenic sinuses were poorly evaluable. Because of the risk of ARDS, fluid resuscitation has been kept lower than a 70% TBSA burn patient would necessitate.

During the hospitalization, several cutaneous swabs were performed and intravenous antibiotic treatment was changed based on antibiograms.

Blood and plasma were transfused routinely both during surgery and hospitalization.

Medical treatment of burn patients and COVID-19 patients shows an overlap.

Treatment with LMWH is mandatory because both burn condition and COVID-19 infection increase the risk of thrombosis.

Significant inflammation is present in patients with SARS-CoV-2 infection. There is the elevation of IL-6 levels, C-reactive protein, erythrocyte sedimentation rate, and fibrinogen. Since the tropism of the virus is for ACE2 receptors, this determines endothelial cell activation and disruption of the antithrombotic state [26].

Broad-spectrum intravenous antibiotics are administered both for the increased risk of sepsis in burn patients and prophylactically in COVID-19 patients to avoid opportunistic infections.

Besides this treatment, which is common in burn patients and COVID-19 patients, she also received specific treatment for COVID-19 pneumonia. In order to improve her ventilation, she was set in a prone position leading to a slow improvement of her gas exchanges [27]. The change to prone position generates a more even distribution of the gas–tissue ratios and a more homogeneous distribution of lung stress and strain. It is also accompanied by an improvement in arterial blood gases, due to a better overall ventilation/perfusion matching [3].

It was then started endovenous corticosteroid therapy, with the goal of improving gas exchanges. Corticosteroid therapy given to COVID-19 patients could have a favorable effect by reducing pro-inflammatory cytokines, decreasing lung vascular permeability, improving epithelial barrier integrity, and promoting alveolar oedema fluid clearance [28].

The patient also started medical treatment with Chloroquine/hydroxychloroquine *(CQ/HCQ)*. Possible mechanisms of action of HCQ are multiple and not fully understood. It probably reduces viral entrance by increasing endosomal pH and inhibits glycosylation of the cellular ACE2 receptor, interfering with viral binding in the lungs [29].

On the twelfth day of hospitalization, her swabs and BALs were negative and the patient showed no more COVID-19 positivities until her last day of hospitalization.

After the negativization of two consequent BALs, the patient was transferred to a non-COVID-19 ICU, according to the fact that her clinical conditions required ICU treatment. In fact, she stayed feverish with temperature oscillating in a range from 37.5°C and 39°C, her chest x-rays showed pleural effusion and her blood tests revealed an overall augmentation of inflammatory parameters.

During the hospitalization, her general conditions were initially quite stable but she slowly developed a septic status, which led the patient to death on her 105th day of recovery.

From a surgical point of view, the day after the hospitalization the patient underwent a massive surgical debridement of all burned areas based on removal of proteolytic enzymes where applied and surgical necrectomy in other areas followed by homologous skin grafting and a total body change of dressing.

Frequent change of dressings in a dedicated operating room was planned (three times a week) and the patient underwent several surgical debridements and homologous and autologous skin grafting procedures.

In order to avoid long-term intubation complications, on the 5th day after hospitalization a tracheostomy was performed.

During hospitalization, we assisted to a gradual re-epithelialization of the burned area, with total healing of her upper left limb but the permanence of not fully healed areas on her chest and dorsum.

Our second COVID-19 positive patient was a 73-year-old man who set himself on fire with turpentine once he found out that his wife had contracted COVID-19 infection. His medical history included blood hypertension, diabetes, and depression.

The patient lived in Bergamo, one of the worst-hit cities by COVID-19 in Italy. He immediately was transferred to his city ER, where he was stabilized, intubated and a BAL was performed with a positive result. The day after, May 7th 2020, he was transported by helicopter to our dedicated operating room, where a new BAL was performed.

He had II and III degree circumferential burns on his lower limbs, III degree burns on the perineum and scrotum, III degree burns on the half of the flanks, chest, and left side of the back, III degree burns on half neck and upper limb with a TBSA of 60%.

The patient was immediately transfused with plasma and underwent double decompressive fasciotomies on his right lower limb. Then surgical and enzymatic debridement was performed on all third-degree burns.

The patient was then transferred to our COVID-19 ICU.

As he showed no COVID-19 symptoms, no pneumonia, and initial negative BAL, a BAL per day was repeated for the next three days and all of them resulted negative. It was also performed a serological test that showed high IgG levels and low IgM levels, a sign of a previous positivity.

As his clinical condition required an ICU, the patient stayed in our COVID-19 ICU, even though he did not develop a COVID-19 infection, and never contracted it during his hospitalization in COVID-19 ICU.

In his hospitalization in COVID-19 ICU, the patient was set on an air fluidized bed (Clinitron®) as adjuvant therapy for his back burns, and standard treatment for burn patient was started: hydration with Ringer lactate's solution for the first 24 hours, then with rehydration solution, antithrombotic therapy with LMWH, broad-spectrum intravenous antibiotics according to microbial cultures, Immunoglobulin therapy for three days (Pentaglobin®) and antalgic therapy.

His vital parameters were monitored, water balance was kept positive, and specific parenteral alimentation rich in proteins and oligo-elements was started.

Routine blood tests and x-rays were made and various microbiological samples were sent.

Thanks to the ICU care we assisted in a gradual recovery of vital parameters, stabilization of the hemodynamic system, and the restoration of spontaneous breathing.

From a respiratory point of view, the patient has been intubated until the 15th of May, when a tracheostomy was performed and he was ventilated through it. Since the 28th of June, he has been spontaneously breathing.

Hemodynamically he required therapy with norepinephrine for about one month.

His recovery in COVID-19 ICU, which in the meantime returned to a non-COVID-19 ICU as the first wave of COVID-19 was about to end, lasted 52 days and then he was transferred to our Burn Unit.

During his hospitalization in our Burn Unit, we assisted in gradual healing and re-epithelialization of all burned areas and the patient was going to be transferred to the Burn Centre of his belonging region for the continuation of treatment.

On the 19th of August the patient complained of dyspnea, he had a fever (41°C) which did not respond to antipyretics. His saturation was 86% with 6 L/min of 02, his blood pressure was 72/32 mmHg, heath rate 105 bpm, and respiratory rate 42 breaths per minute. A septic shock was developing. He was immediately transferred to the ICU and intubated but he died some days later because of the worsening of the septic shock.

It is clear that death in this patient is related to the severity of his burns and not to COVID-19.

Nevertheless, this case remarks once again how fundamental is the management of a COVID-19 burn patient since the beginning, with the use of a dedicated operating room and the recovery in a COVID-19 ICU.

In the month of October 2020, all of Italy was affected by the second wave of COVID-19, with the viral spread and the crescent burden on ICUs. This led to the diffusion of the infection inside the hospitals and the genesis of clusters of infection.

As a matter of fact, between October 8th and November 30th 2020, two of our patients got infected by the virus several weeks after their hospitalization.

Thanks to our protocol, which contemplates the repetition of antigenic and molecular COVID-19 swabs weekly, we managed to identify and immediately isolate patients affected by COVID-19, in order to reduce the spread of infection inside our Burn Unit.

None of our patients who contracted the infection showed any COVID-19-like symptoms. They had only a mild fever, which wasn't imputable to the virus. In fact, all of them had a mild augmentation of inflammatory parameters and microbiological growth (*Pseudomonas aeruginosa* above all) on their burns. In fact, fever is one of the most frequent symptoms in burn patients.

It is curious that they had their first positive molecular swab on the 8th of October and continued to alternate positive and negative molecular swabs until the 30th of November.

These patients never showed any significant symptoms and had been isolated in a single room for all the positivity period. Further examinations were made, in fact, a sputum culture examination was performed and within approximately one week we had the result: no SARS-CoV-2 growth. So all the molecular swabs which resulted positive after the sputum examination were false positive and the patients were not considered contagious anymore.

Until an effective circumscription of positive cases has been achieved, it was taken the hard decision not to hospitalize other burn patients which did not come, of course, from our ER.

Spatial isolation, the use of PPE, the weekly screening program, and the disinfection of all common spaces were fundamental to circumscribe the COVID-19 cluster which was born in our Burn Unit.

Once safety was finally achieved it was restarted regular hospitalization, always according to our COVID-19 protocol.

The third COVID-19 burn patient was a 51-year-old female who burned her face due to a backfire, reporting only II-degree burns. At the arrival, an ENT consultation was made and it stated intubation wasn't necessary. A molecular swab was made and it tested positive for COVID-19. The patient was completely asymptomatic and was hospitalized in our Burn Unit.

She underwent surgical debridement and an amniotic membrane grafting was performed. Her hospitalization lasted for 6 days and then she was dismissed.

Our last burn patient affected by COVID-19 was a 25-year-old female.

She had contracted the infection ten days before the burn and she was in home isolation, as her conditions did not require hospitalization. Her home treatment included antipyretics, Azithromycin once a day for six days, no LMWH or corticosteroids were necessary. No other significant medical history was reported.

Due to this injury, she reported second-degree burns on her neck and cheeks; third-degree burns circumferential on her upper limbs, second-degree on her chest and breasts; second-degree on her abdomen with a TBSA of 41%. We decided to immediately perform enzymatic debridement with Nexobrid® (**Figure 1**), and after 24 hours we performed coverage within homologous skin grafts and amniotic membrane. The patient was then transferred to a COVID-19 ICU.

During her hospitalization in ICU, she did not present any COVID-19-like symptoms and her BALs negativized five days after her hospitalization, so no specific treatment for COVID-19 was started and she received standard therapy for burn patients. In two weeks the patient was stabilized and transferred to our Burn Unit and her skin injuries were definitely closed by an autologous skin graft.

This case series reported how the novel SARS-CoV-2 afflicted our Burn Unit and how we managed to adapt our Burn Unit admission because of the pandemic. It is important to underline that none of our patients affected by COVID-19 ever developed interstitial pneumonia and so COVID-19 infection did not directly influence the outcome of our patients.

What actually was influenced by the pandemic was the management of the patient, the preparation of the operating room, and the surgical act itself.

2.3 Surgical treatment of Sars-CoV-2 patients

For most burn patients coming to the OR, the need for surgical intervention is imperative. Patients urgently admitted to any Burn Unit generally need immediate transfer to the OR for the primary care of their wounds and, mostly, will need subsequent surgical reassessments and re-interventions until an acceptable cover of the wounds has been achieved and the patient may be followed up as an outpatient.

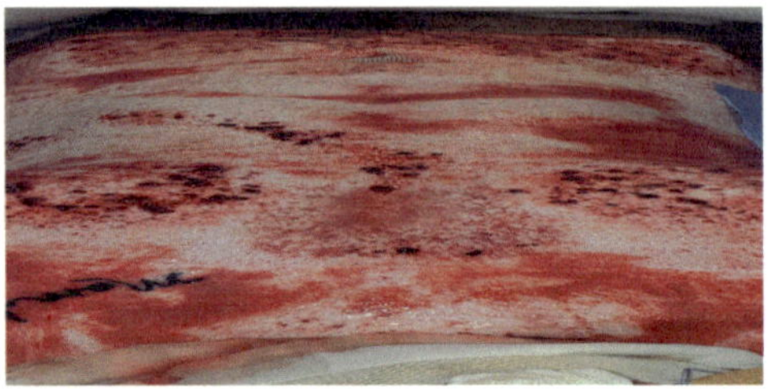

Figure 1.
Third degree burn abdoment and chest 4 hour after enzimatic debridment with Nexobrid.

The urgent admission and the subsequent surgical revisions expose medical personnel involved in burned patient care to an increased risk of contracting SARS-CoV-2 due to prolonged exposure in the OR and in the Burn Unit itself. Besides, the exposure risk also applies to the other patients admitted to the OR or the wards due to proximity.

As vaccine rollout proceeds, more and more people are getting immunized to SARS-CoV-2, however, as vaccination efforts are still underway, screening at admission, isolation protocols for positive patients and safe surgical and anesthesiologic procedures for the personnel are still to be enforced to ensure spread avoidance.

In our experience, the protocol enforced to screen SARS-CoV-2 patients entering our ward has worked fine in avoiding admission of positive patients and in avoiding spreading of the infection among inpatients and to or from healthcare workers [17].

In general, struggling with a pandemic and having hospitals overwhelmed by SARS-CoV-2 positive patients in various degrees of severity, required careful organization, and eventual re-organization, of the health care staff activity from nurses to medical doctors to support personnel in order to avoid exhaustion of resources. This is especially true for surgical equipment which cannot be easily replaced with new, less trained staff or by staff taken from other branches of medicine without the risk of reducing senior surgical expertise hence the standard of care. From here, the need to work on skeleton personnel in order to spare as many units as possible in case of health care personnel contagion. In general, this type of approach has been required to minimize almost all elective surgical activities and to postpone them to the moment when contagion levels start, slowly, to reduce in number. The only elective patients that kept on being admitted were the oncological ones and only after submission of a negative SARS-CoV-2 RT- PCR test dated no more than 3 days before admission. However, obviously, emergent patients did not disappear during COVID-19 pandemic and their management has been the greatest concern of all in order to guarantee assistance, but to avoid excessive personnel exposure.

In Italy, the major medical societies involved in the care of surgical patients have produced indications for the management of potential SARS-CoV-2 patients [30] which often are the backbone of each hospital-specific protocol.

As the emergent need for surgery does not allow time to wait for SARS-CoV-2 swab results, all patients admitted in emergency must be treated as if they were positive.

As, usually, transport is needed to bring the patient from the ward or from elsewhere to the theater, clear and pre-designed pathways should be available. These paths should be the shortest possible and the most isolated possible, as this is clearly not always possible, anyone crossing these paths should be alerted preemptively or these paths should be cleared before passage and sanitized afterwards. Transport personnel should be trained to wear appropriate PPE at all times.

In general, patients going to theater should not stop anywhere for any reason but should be brought to the designated theater where all procedures pre, peri, and post-operational should be performed and that designated theater should be the one closest to theater entry in order to minimize transit contagion risk. Entry and exit pathways to the theater should be different from negative patients' routes. Potentially positive patients should wear the protective masks until anesthesiologic procedures for tubing begin, otherwise, if there is no need for intubation, the protective mask should be worn at all times. Clearly, the personnel that will care for the patient, needs to be trained in donning, doffing, and in the disposal of protective equipment (**Figure 2**).

In the OR minimal personnel should be allocated to a single infected case in order to minimize exposure and, if the case spans more than one shift, this could mean working after hours for the equipment involved. All personnel receiving the

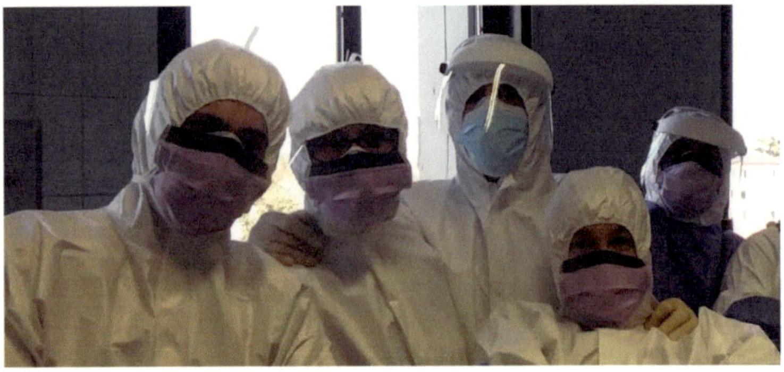

Figure 2.
Preparation to a Covid burned patient surgery with all protective disposable.

patient should be wearing appropriate PPE. All non-necessary material must remain outside the OR including medical records which may be consulted either by doffing or by personnel non involved in the OR and then communicated inside the OR.

OR should be negative-pressurized with a high air exchange cycle rate. Materials available should be ready on a case-by-case basis before the procedure begins and, once it starts, all efforts should be made to use what is available in order to reduce to the least possible entry and exit of personnel to and from the OR. All trolleys should be replaced with dedicated ones in order to avoid possible surface contagion for procedures to come afterwards. Personnel must be reduced to the minimum number possible to perform the planned operation.

Anesthesiologists should have planned their strategy in advance in order to minimize risks associated with complex intubation procedures and techniques with the highest chance of first-time success should be used to reduce excessive manipulation of the airways. All staff must wear full PPE and these should be replaced after completing the procedure, especially if that has been complex.

More liberal use of intubation is acceptable to avoid risks associated with non-invasive ventilation. RSI could potentially reduce the need for manual ventilation and potential aerosol spreading, which could however be reduced by using small current volumes in manual ventilation. HEPA filters should be put between the patient's expiratory limb and the ventilator machine and between the patient and the gas sampling tube and replaced after each use.

As all materials should be ready before the procedure starts, all efforts must be made to use the material available. Entering or exiting the room should be discouraged at all times. Any need for additional material should be addressed by personnel outside the OR. Surgical masks are replaced by FFP2 all the remaining donning should be performed as protocols indicate. The patient is dressed according to the procedure to be performed.

For what concerns the procedure, no consensus exists on whether laparoscopy should be used or should be contraindicated [31]. There is the theoretical possibility of spreading the virus through smoke produced by energy devices, but this has not been demonstrated for SARS-CoV-2. The same applies to energy devices used in open surgery. No formal contraindication exists to perform laparoscopic procedures in SARS-CoV-2 patients either positive or suspected, however, all precautions must be applied to reduce potential exposures including reducing the use of electrosurgical devices, applying smoke evacuators and HEPA filters to exhaustion of surgical smoke, reducing pneumoperitoneum pressures [32] and, finally, deflating the abdomen using suction or smoke evacuation devices instead of letting pneumoperitoneum out from trocar incisions in the OR [33].

Otherwise, we need to perform a protection colostomy for burn legs in our second COVID-19 patient and we preferred to perform it by open laparotomy due to efforts to avoid gas diffusion on COVID-19 tissues and the presence of abundant abdomen's free liquid [34].

After the procedure, enough time should be allowed for air exchange in the OR according to the exchange cycle rate of the theater to avoid cross-contamination. All environments in which the patient has transited should be carefully sanitized. All waste should be disposed of in designated containers and should transported wearing full PPE.

2.4 Burned patient swab surveillance

Screening swabs on the healthcare workers were scheduled weekly while on hospitalized patients twice a week. In the first 6 months from the beginning of the pandemic, no outbreak occurred in the ward, neither among staff nor among patients.

For scheduled surgical interventions instead, a telephone triage was performed to find out if in the previous 2 weeks the patient had developed any symptoms compatible with a possible COVID-19 infection, such as fever, cough, breathing difficulties, asthenia, anosmia, or ageusia. If the patient did not report any symptoms or known positive contacts, molecular swabs were performed in the 96-72 h before hospitalization, requiring the patient to be isolated at home after the execution [16].

In early October, rapid antigenic swabs began to be used mainly by the infectious disease department and the emergency room. During the second week of October a small Coronavirus outbreak involving two healthcare workers as well as two patients, developed inside the Burn Unit. This led to the request to the infectious diseases department for a supply of rapid antigenic swabs, to obtain a faster and more efficient screening of patients and medical staff.

Up to that time, the standard hospital procedure, in case of unprotected contact with a patient positive for COVID-19, included the execution of a molecular swab: immediately after contact, on the 5th and the 10th day.

During this screening period, the operator, if asymptomatic and tested negative, was not required to stay in home isolation.

The main problem with this screening routine based on molecular swabs was the report timing. In fact, at that time, a screening swab, given the large amount of work to which the laboratory was subjected, was rarely reported before 2–3 days.

These timing of execution, considering the incubation period and the high percentage of asymptomatic patients with the COVID-19 infection, subjected the staff, who had to work daily with positive patients, to a concrete risk, if they had contracted the virus, to act as vectors before the swabs detected their positivity.

To reduce this risk, we decided that the screening for the viral detection in the major burn centre had to be carried out by performing a double swab: antigenic and molecular at the same time.

Although at that time many studies had already reported an antigenic swabs sensitivity varying between 30% and 80%, considerably inferior compared to the molecular swabs one, reported around 97%, the speed of execution made it possible to anticipate possible isolation by a few days, thus reducing the possibility of any intra-hospital infections and the onset of new outbreaks [35–37].

With the double swab method, screenings continued to be carried out every 7 days on healthcare workers, twice a week (usually on Monday and Friday) on hospitalized patients, at 0–5-10 days for unprotected contacts and as needed for personnel or patients who presented suggestive symptoms such as fever, arthralgia, anosmia or malaise.

The "double-swab" screening continued till the end of February when the healthcare workers got vaccinated. From that moment, weekly, only molecular swabs are performed, while "double-swabs" screening is still carried out nowadays for unvaccinated hospitalized patients.

From the beginning of this double swab protocol, no patient got infected during their hospitalization. We registered four cases of SARS-CoV-2 infection between healthcare personnel, all of them immediately quarantined with none of them contracting the infection in the workplace.

3. Therapeutic consideration in a COVID-19 burn patient

Burn-injured patients are deeply affected in nearly all their vital functions with pathophysiologic changes that can range from hemodynamic instability to altered metabolism, hypothermia, and, more importantly, airway and pulmonary impaired functions.

SARS-CoV-2 has represented in Italy an impressive public health threat, rapidly spreading among regions with Lombardy and Veneto as epidemic centres. Because of the high viral infectious rate and its capability to damage several organs, especially the lung with particular severe pneumonia, effective prevention and treatment are essential [12].

Various treatment options are being tested, with a variety of studies investigating the utility of some off-label drugs. Currently, the major way to avoid virus spreading is epidemiologic control through preventive measures such as isolation of infected patients and identification of the source of infection. All categories of people are susceptible to SARS-CoV-2 but most severe cases are recognized in the elderly patients and those with underlying diseases or immune dysfunctions [6, 13]. Burn injuries must be considered similar to the above-mentioned conditions for their intrinsic immune and multiple organ dysregulation, in the context of a general severe illness affecting all vital functions [14].

The fast COVID-19 spread from China to European countries such as Italy, and particularly the region in which our centre is located, therefore imperatively required the implementation of every procedure and admission protocol in our Burn Unit.

COVID-19 treatment guidelines are continuously updating based on revising, legitimate national and international guidelines for optimal management. Antivirals such as Kaletra, Favipiravir and Remdesivir have been used by infectious disease consultants but are not part of our COVID-19 treatment guidelines yet. Oseltamivir or Ribavirin are not used any longer. Hydroxychloroquine has not been used anymore in the treatment of COVID-19 patients.

Interferon-Beta and/or IVIG have been given in case of excessive inflammatory responses, mostly in our burn critical care COVID-19 patients. Corticosteroids such as Dexamethasone and Methyl-prednisolone have recently been added to our COVID-19 treatment protocols in the setting of severe inflammatory responses and/or hypoxemia (blood oxygen saturation < 90%). Convalescent plasma has also been added to the therapeutic regimen of deteriorating burn critical care cases. All our adult patients (ward or ICU, with or without COVID-19) have been receiving pharmacological thromboprophylaxis (low molecular weight Heparin, standard-dose unfractionated Heparin) unless there were contraindications.

Frequent use of antibiotics without clear indications is not anymore recommended. However, they have often been used in burn critical care cases with worsening clinical conditions. All our patients receive the usual dose of daily vitamin C, per standard burn treatment protocols. Our current COVID-19 guidelines have not yet recommended high dose vitamin C.

Concomitant severe burn and COVID-19 might complicate the clinical presentation and hospital course.

This dictates multidisciplinary approaches to risk stratify, screen, assess, and manage coexisting diseases. Additionally, appropriate preparations and careful precautions need to be executed in burn units to prevent COVID-19 exposure and transmission to limit potential adverse outcomes.

The potential detrimental consequences of concomitant burn and COVID-19 suggest mandating extra precautions and sophisticated strategies which need to be implemented in burn units. Such policies help prevent infection, recognize different types of exposure, establish detailed and systematic protocols on proper diagnosis and management. The key steps include the fast and careful patient screening for COVID-19 on arrival, frequent screening of hospital staff, obtaining detailed history on travel risk factors in two weeks prior to the admission, assess for fever or other respiratory signs and symptoms before or during hospitalization with continuous clinical surveillance, personal protective equipment (PPE) in all areas with proper social distancing, provision of disinfectants and sanitation equipment, and staff travel restrictions [15, 16].

With an ongoing COVID-19 pandemic, SARS-CoV-2 infection might be a preceding, concomitant, or subsequent disease in addition to other various medical problems or traumas such as burns. Thorough risk stratification and multidisciplinary approaches to the strategic management of comorbid conditions are paramount to prevent possible worsening outcomes.

Current evidence demonstrated sensitivity rates of less than 70% for all COVID-19 diagnostic tests including RNA RT-PCR, total antibody, IgM, and IgG at the first week of symptom onset. In addition, the test-positive result rates of RNA RT-PCR tests (currently the most performed test in the UK) varies depending on the sampling technique (eg. oropharyngeal swab, NP swab, bronchoalveolar lavage) and timing of the test from symptom onset significant presence of false-negative tests should always be taken into consideration pending the development of validated, highly sensitive and specific tests.

All healthcare workers and patients should attempt to deliver care whilst ensuring protection from disease transmission by any means available. All burns services should anticipate and plan to continue delivering patient care whilst taking social distancing and shielding measures into account.

The shocking speed with which the COVID-19 pandemic has exploded, and the scale of strategic planning required to cope make it very difficult for systems to prepare adequately. In many places, the critical care demand will create sudden scarcity which will impact the capacity to provide critical care for burns. This obligates each burn centre to prepare for burn care under austere conditions. In cases of massive COVID-19 disease, the burn centre will become an important cache of personnel, space, and equipment. Burn centre leadership should actively engage in local and regional strategic planning. Importantly, the burn community should seek ways to help one another through the coming challenge. The present collection of experiences aims to achieve the goal of early communication among burn leaders in order to disseminate knowledge rapidly and fast-track best practices.

SARS-CoV-2 screening and prevention strategies need to be implemented at burn care centres, both outpatient and inpatient settings during the current COVID-19 pandemic. This is due to the substantial vulnerability of burn casualties to infection and the ease of transmission among them.

The effectiveness of the adopted measures during the COVID-19 epidemic outburst allowed our Burn Unit to preserve its clinical and surgical activity simultaneously safeguarding patients and hospital personnel from contagion risk, despite a high rate of admitted critical patients and the geographical position in the centre of an epidemic area.

3.1 Medical and surgical approach in the COVID-19 burn patient

Medical treatment of burn patients and COVID-19 patients show an overlap. The low number of treated cases could not allow any consideration about the absence of COVID-19 complications in burned patients. At the same time, we have to underline that several therapeutic approaches that seemed to improve Sars-CoV-2 affected patients are common to severely burned patients.

- **Low molecular weight heparin**: Treatment with LMWH is mandatory because both burn condition and COVID-19 infection increase the risk of thrombosis.

  Significant inflammation is present in patients with SARS-CoV-2 infection. There is the elevation of IL-6 levels, C-reactive protein, and erythrocyte sedimentation rate, and fibrinogen.

  Since the tropism of the virus is for ACE2 receptors, this determines endothelial cell activation and disruption of the antithrombotic state [2].

- **Antibiotic treatment**: Broad-spectrum intravenous antibiotics are administered both for the increased risk of sepsis in burn patients and prophylactically in COVID-19 patients to avoid opportunistic infections.

- **Plasma transfusion:** Plasma transfusion is a life-saving and fundamental treatment in burn patients because it represents the best resuscitation fluid due to its capability to restore intravascular volume status and treat the endotheliopathy. Hyperimmune plasma from COVID-19 convalescent was also suggested as a potential treatment for severe COVID-19 so, even though we have not experienced such treatment in our cases, it could be possible to consider the treatment of burn patients with severe SARS-CoV-2 infection by hyperimmune plasma.

- **Immunoglobulin:** Depressed serum immunoglobulin levels following severe burns may lead to subsequent infectious complications following such injuries so the administration of immunoglobulin in our therapeutic approach in major burns is common (*Pentaglobin®* at 100 ml rate three times a day for three days). At the same time immunomodulation with polyclonal preparation of immunoglobulins as adjuvant therapy in SARS-CoV-2 mild and severe pneumonia has been detected as efficacy in several cases [38, 39].

  At the same time about the medical approach, we have to emphasize the mismatch between the important fluid resuscitation necessary for burn patients and the fluid restriction that is needed in SARS-CoV-2 pneumonia.

  In the surgical approach to COVID-19 burned patients we have marked some important aspects to be considered:

- **Necrectomy approach:** Due to the necessity to reduce operating time and at the same time to be efficient with necrectomy we increased the use of enzymatic debridement (*Nexobrid* ®- Mediwound Germany GmbH) which allows an efficient and selective debridement with less blood loss [40].

- **Hydrodebridement:** We have avoided the use of hydro-debridement (such Versajet®) for wound bed preparation due to the necessity to have not spreading of virus particles into operating theater and on objects

- **Laparoscopic procedures:** When laparoscopic procedures were necessary (eg. Protection colostomy) we avoided performing because of the high risk of contamination with the insufflate air and we preferred the laparotomy approach

- **Tracheostomy:** To perform a tracheostomy on COVID-19 patients it's necessary a well-trained and experienced surgeon with a strict collaboration with an anesthesiologist in all parts of the procedure, in particular, to avoid any air spreading from the tube.

- **Personnel and equipment:** Personnel must be reduced to the minimum possible number with a very precise surgical planning. The equipment must be the same as in the COVID-19 ward unit and because of the high temperature needed during burn patient operations and the physical efforts, it's mandatory to perform early surgical procedures.

- **Pathways:** Dedicate pathways must be planned for COVID-19 positive patients from and to the OR and must be separated from regular pathways for non-COVID-19 patients.

- **Air circulation and operating room preparation:** Air circulation has to be achieved by using dedicated filters and numerous air exchanges. The OR must be equipped with the minimum instruments available and with easily sterilized tools, as it needs accurate disinfection after every procedure.

4. Conclusion

In the early weeks of the pandemic, with the first cluster of cases detected on 21th and 22th of February and a national quarantine declared on March 8th, the Italian National Health System found itself in a very stressful situation, counting a high number of the greatest number of cases and deaths and requiring an intense effort to secure bed availability in the hospitals and the ICUs.

Even if our elective activity was reduced to the correction of burn sequelae, urgent and emergent activities greatly increased since many other centres in North Italy could not accept burn patients anymore due to ICU bed lacking or furthermore for incapability to accept and treat COVID 19 positive patients.

To avoid a possible spreading of SARS-CoV-2 inside the Burn Unit, and to reduce the risk patients and health workers were submitted to, since the beginning of the emergency period we developed a protocol for the acceptance of all the new patients and the surveillance of the hospitalized ones [17].

This protocol was elaborated gathering guidelines and suggestions reported by the first Burn Centers involved in COVID-19 infection management [41, 42]. It anticipated the general prevention and management indications established by the Medical Direction of the University Hospital of Padua, which followed the most updated Italian Government and International literature guidelines at the time [18, 19].

Three principles are the pillars of this protocol: patients' history (suggestive symptoms or contact with cases are themself sufficient causes for isolation, even if the test performed is negative), rapid testing, and isolation in a dedicated room until the test response.

Our Burn Unit Centre is a third level facility, responsible for the acceptance and treatment of all major burns in an area with a population of approximately 5 million people. When the response timing did not interfere with the urgent treatment, we asked the patient to be tested by the sending hospital or by our emergency room.

For emergency cases instead, with major burns, our microbiological lab granted us a preferential route to obtain the results of the swabs within 90 minutes, while the patients were kept in isolation in a quarantine room or the operatory room if intubated, before being moved to the Ward, semi-ICU or ICU according to their conditions.

While since the beginning of the epidemic we decided to stop any outside visits to inpatient rooms, encouraging the use of phone or video calls to communicate with relatives, an exemption was made for pediatric cases, where the caregiver was tested simultaneously with the child or as soon as he arrived, staying in the monitoring room till the swab's result.

The nucleic acid detection through reverse transcription qualitative PCR was the only method accepted for the laboratory diagnosis, usually via the collection of nasal and pharyngeal swabs but also via BAL in ventilated patients, which proved to be a more sensible detector [43].

Once confirmed negative, the patients are finally moved to the Burn Unit strictly monitored for 14 days as recommended by the World Health Organization (WHO) [44].

Considering no SARS-CoV-2 outbreak has happened in our Burn Unit since the beginning of the double testing, despite the second wave of COVID-19 Italy has experienced from November 2020, we can consider it an appropriate way of managing SARS-CoV-2 screening on hospitalized patients and healthcare workers.

COVID-19 infection in burn patients might worsen the clinical outcome making medical care, even more, demanding, with the necessity of multidisciplinary care.

Management of surgical patients affected or potentially affected by SARS-CoV-2 requires clear protocols that must be shared with health care staff in order to be implemented. Careful observation of safety rules must be present at all times to avoid infection spread. All non-emergency procedures should be postponed until a negative RT-PCR test is available for the patient. Clearly, every measure is work-demanding and requires very high compliance to the rules applied, however, following protocols will be the only way to go back to normal activity in the shortest time possible.

Currently, the development of at least 7 different vaccines based on 3 platforms and their entry into the market represents the best hope for the global population to reach the herd immunity necessary to stop the viral spread.

The mass vaccination program started in December 2020. Despite clinical trials presenting high levels of efficacy of several COVID-19 vaccines, like all other vaccines, they will not be completely effective.

The development of other variants resistant to immunization and how many people get vaccinated are just a few of the possible variants to be included in the complex evaluation of the global success of the vaccination process.

Conflict of interest

Publication cost was supported by MediWound Ltd. Company.

Abbreviations

COVID-19	coronavirus disease 2019
SARS-CoV-2	severe acute respiratory syndrome coronavirus 2
ARDS	acute respiratory distress syndrome
ICU	intensive care unit
BU	Burn Unit

OR	operation room
CT	computer tomography
BAL	broncho-alveolar lavage
RT-PCR	real time polymerase chain reaction
TBSA	total body surface area
ER	emergency room
PPE	personal protection equipment

Author details

Filippo Andrea Giovanni Perozzo[1*], Alex Pontini[1*], Alberto De Lazzari[1], Alvise Montanari[1], Giovanni Valotto[2] and Bruno Azzena[1]

1 Burn and Plastic Surgery Unit, Padua University Hospital, Padua, Italy

2 1st General Surgery Unit , Padua University Hospital, Padua, Italy

*Address all correspondence to: filippo.perozzo@gmail.com
and alex.pontini@aopd.veneto.it

References

[1] Li Q., Guan X., Wu P., Wang X., Zhou L., Tong Y. Early transmission dynamics in Wuhan, China, of novel coronavirus-infected pneumonia. *N Engl J Med.* 2020;382:1199-1207. doi: 10.1056/NEJMoa2001316.

[2] Liu Y., Gayle A.A., Wilder-Smith A., Rocklöv J. The reproductive number of COVID-19 is higher compared to SARS coronavirus. *J Travel Med.* 2020;27 doi: 10.1093/jtm/taaa021.

[3] Fu Y, Cheng Y, Wu Y. Understanding SARS-CoV-2-mediated inflammatory responses: from mechanisms to potential therapeutic tools. Virol Sin 2020;35(3):266-71. https://doi.org/10.1007/s12250-020-00207-4.

[4] Lu C.W., Liu X.F., Jia Z.F. 2019-nCoV transmission through the ocular surface must not be ignored. *Lancet.* 2020;395(February (10224)) doi: 10.1016/S0140-6736(20)30313-5. [PMC free article] [PubMed] [CrossRef] [Google Scholar]

[5] Carlos W.G., Dela Cruz C.S., Cao B., Pasnick S., Jamil S. Novel Wuhan (2019-nCoV) coronavirus m. *J Respir Crit Care Med.* 2020;201 doi: 10.1164/rccm.2014P7. [PubMed] [CrossRef] [Google Scholar

[6] Gheblawi M, Wang K, Viveiros A, Nguyen Q, Zhong J-C, Turner AJ, Raizada MK,Grant MB, Oudit GY. Angiotensin-converting enzyme 2: SARS-CoV-2 receptorand regulator of the renin-angiotensin system: celebrating the 20thanniversary of the discovery of ACE2. Circ Res 2020;126(10):1456-74. https://doi.org/10.1161/CIRCRESAHA.120.317015.

[7] Feng J-Y, Chien J-Y, Kao K-C, Tsai C-L, Hung FM, Lin F-M, Hu H-C, Huang K-L, YuC-J, Yang K-Y. Predictors of early onset multiple organ dysfunction in major burn patients with ventilator support: experience from a mass casualty explosion. Sci Rep 2018;8(1). https://doi.org/10.1038/s41598-018-29158-3.

[8] Herndon DN, Tompkins RG. Support of the metabolic response to burn injury. Lancet 2004;363(9424):1895-902. https://doi.org/10.1016/S0140-6736(04)16360-5.

[9] Hesamirostami M, Nazarian R, Asghari H, et al. A case series of concomitant burn and COVID-19. *Burns Open*. 2021;5(1):34-38. doi:10.1016/j.burnso.2020.11.003

[10] Accardo-Palumbo A, D'Amelio L, Pileri D, D'Arpa N, Mogavero R, Amato G, et al.Reduction of plasma granzyme A correlates with severity of sepsis in burn patients. Burns2010;36(6):811-8. https://doi.org/10.1016/j.burns.2009.11.009.

[11] Smith DL, Cairns BA, Ramadan F, Dalston JS, Fakhry SM, Rutledge R, Meyer AA,Peterson HD. Effect of inhalation injury, burn size, and age on mortality: a study of 1447 consecutive burn patients. J Trauma 1994;37(4):655-9. https://doi.org/10.1097/00005373-199410000-00021.

[12] Lorente JA, Vallejo A, Galeiras R, Tómicic V, Zamora J, Cerdá E, de la Cal MA,Esteban A. Organ dysfunction as estimated by the sequential organ failure assessment score is related to outcome in critically ill burn patients. Shock2009;31(2):125-31. https://doi.org/10.1097/SHK.0b013e31817fc3ef.

[13] Huang C., Wang Y., Li X., Ren L., Zhao J., Hu Y. Clinical features of patients infected with 2019 novel coronavirus in Wuhan, China. *Lancet.* 2020;395 doi: 10.1016/S0140-6736(20)30183-30185.

[14] Chen G., Wu D., Guo W., Cao Y., Huang D., Wang H. Clinical and

immunological features of severe and moderate coronavirus disease 2019. *J Clin Invest.* 2020;130(May (5)):2620-2629. doi: 10.1172/JCI137244.

[15] Wu Yi-Chi, Chen Ching-Sung, Chan Yu-Jiun. The outbreak of COVID-19: an overview. *J Chin Med Assoc.* 2020;83(March (3)):217-220. doi: 10.1097/JCMA.0000000000000270. [PMC free article] [PubMed] [CrossRef] [Google Scholar]

[16] Facchin F., Scarpa C., Vindigni V., Bassetto F. Effectiveness of preventive measures against Covid-19 in a Plastic Surgery Unit in the epicenter of the pandemic in Italy Plastic and Reconstructive Surgery. *Plast Reconstr Surg.* 2020;(April):332-333. doi: 10.1016/j.hansur.2020.04.007. [PubMed] [CrossRef] [Google Scholar]

[17] Azzena B, Perozzo FAG, De Lazzari A, Valotto G, Pontini A. Burn Unit admission and management protocol during COVID-19 pandemic. *Burns*. 2021;47(1):52-57. doi:10.1016/j.burns.2020.09.004

[18] Covid-19, Raccomandazioni per gli operatori sanitari. Available: http://www.salute.gov.it/portale/nuovocoronavirus/dettaglioContenutiNuovoCoronavirus.jsp?lingua=italiano&id=5373&area=nuovoCoronavirus&menu=vuoto#5. [Accessed: 31 May 2020].

[19] CDC. Information for healthcare professionals about coronavirus (COVID-19) CDC. Available: https://www.cdc.gov/coronavirus/2019-nCoV/hcp/index.html. [Accessed: 31 May 2020].

[20] Infection prevention and control during health care when novel coronavirus (nCoV) infection is suspected. Available: https://www.who.int/publications-detail/infection-prevention-and-control-during-health-care-when-novel-coronavirus-(ncov)-infection-is-suspected-20200125. [Accessed: 31 May 2020].

[21] Huang Z., Zhuang D., Xiong B., Deng D.X., Li H., Lai W. Occupational exposure to SARS-CoV-2 in burns treatment during the COVID-19 epidemic: specific diagnosis and treatment protocol. Biomed Pharmacother. 2020;127(July) Elsevier Masson SAS. - PMC - PubMed

[22] Ağalar C., Öztürk Engin D. Protective measures for covid-19 for healthcare providers and laboratory personnel. Turk J Med Sci. 2020;50 (SI-1):578-584. doi: 10.3906/sag-2004-132. Turkiye Klinikleri. - DOI - PMC - PubMed

[23] European Centre for Disease Prevention and Control . ECDC; Stockholm, Sweden: 2020. Infection prevention and control for COVID-19 in healthcare settings. ECDC technical report. [12 March 2020]

[24] World Health Organization . WHO; Geneva, Switzerland: 2020. Clinical management of severe acute respiratory infection (SARI) when COVID-19 disease is suspected: interim guidance. [13 March 2020]

[25] Lauer S.A., Grantz K.H., Bi Q., Jones F.K., Zheng Q., Meredith H. The incubation period of coronavirus disease 2019 (COVID-19) from publicly reported confirmed cases: estimation and application. Ann Intern Med. 2020;(March):1-7. doi: 10.7326/M20-0504. - DOI - PMC - PubMed

[26] Connors JM, Levy.COVID-19 and its implications for thrombosis and anticoagulation. JH.Blood. 2020 Jun 4;135(23):2033 2040.doi:10.1182/blood.2020006000.PMID: 3233922

[27] Guérin C, Albert RK, Beitler J, Gattinoni L, Jaber S, Marini JJ, Munshi L, Papazian L, Pesenti A,

Vieillard-Baron A, Mancebo J. Prone position in ARDS patients: why, when, how and for whom. Intensive Care Med. 2020 Dec;46(12):2385-2396. doi: 10.1007/s00134-020-06306-w. Epub 2020 Nov 10. PMID: 33169218; PMCID: PMC7652705.

[28] Matthay MA, Wick KD. Corticosteroids, COVID-19 pneumonia, and acute respiratory distress syndrome. J Clin Invest. 2020 Dec 1;130(12):6218-6221. doi:10.1172/JCI143331.PMID: 32976118

[29] Izda V, Jeffries MA, Sawalha AH. COVID-19: A review of therapeutic strategies and vaccine candidates. Clin Immunol. 2021 Jan;222:108634. doi: 10.1016/j.clim.2020.108634. Epub 2020 Nov 17. PMID: 33217545

[30] Coccolini F, Perrone G, Chiarugi M, et al. Surgery in COVID-19 patients : operational directives. 2020;2:1-7.

[31] Simone B De, Chouillard E, Saverio S Di, et al. Emergency surgery during the COVID-19 pandemic : what you need to know for practice. 2020:323-332. doi:10.1308/rcsann.2020.0097

[32] Moletta L, Pierobon ES, Capovilla G, et al. International guidelines and recommendations for surgery during Covid-19 pandemic : A Systematic Review. Int J Surg. 2020;79(May):180-188.

[33] Bordes J, Le R, Bourdais L, Gamelin A. ScienceDirect Perineal burn care : French working group recommendations. 2013;0. doi:10.1016/j.burns.2013.09.007

[34] Ng JWG, Cairns SA, Boyle CPO. ScienceDirect Management of the lower gastrointestinal system in burn : A comprehensive review. 2015;2:0-9. doi:10.1016/j.burns.2015.08.007

[35] Mak GC, Cheng PK, Lau SS, Wong KK, Lau CS, Lam ET, Chan RC, Tsang DN. Evaluation of rapid antigen test for detection of SARS-CoV-2 virus. J Clin Virol. 2020 Aug;129:104500. doi: 10.1016/j.jcv.2020.104500. Epub 2020 Jun 8. PMID: 32585619; PMCID: PMC7278630.

[36] Scohy A, Anantharajah A, Bodéus M, Kabamba-Mukadi B, Verroken A, Rodriguez-Villalobos H. Low performance of rapid antigen detection test as frontline testing for COVID-19 diagnosis. J Clin Virol. 2020 Aug;129:104455. doi: 10.1016/j.jcv.2020.104455. Epub 2020 May 21. PMID: 32485618; PMCID: PMC7240272.

[37] Tsang NNY, So HC, Ng KY, Cowling BJ, Leung GM, Ip DKM. Diagnostic performance of different sampling approaches for SARS-CoV-2 RT-PCR testing: a systematic review and meta-analysis. Lancet Infect Dis. 2021 Apr 12:S1473-3099(21)00146-8. doi: 10.1016/S1473-3099(21)00146-8. Epub ahead of print. PMID: 33857405; PMCID: PMC8041361.

[38] Carannante N, Fiorentino G, Corcione A, et al. Administration of Immunoglobulins in SARS-CoV-2-Positive Patient Is Associated With Fast Clinical and Radiological Healing: Case Report. Frontiers in Medicine. 2020 ;7:388. DOI: 10.3389/fmed.2020.00388. PMID: 32766266; PMCID: PMC7378528.

[39] Bohländer F, Riehl D, Weißmüller S, et al. Immunomodulation: Immunoglobulin Preparations Suppress Hyperinflammation in a COVID-19 Model *via* FcγRIIA and FcαRI. Frontiers in Immunology. 2021;12:700429. DOI: 10.3389/fimmu.2021.700429. PMID: 34177967; PMCID: PMC8223875.

[40] Yew L Loo, Benjamina K L Goh, Steven Jeffery An Overview of the Use of Bromelain-Based Enzymatic Debridement (Nexobrid®) in Deep Partial and Full Thickness Burns: Appraising the Evidence J Burn Care Res 2018 Oct 23;39(6):932-938. doi: 10.1093/jbcr/iry009.

[41] Li Ning, Liu Tingmin, Chen Hualing, Liao Jianmei. Management strategies for the burn ward during COVID-19 pandemic. Burns. 2020;46(June (4)):756-761. doi: 10.1016/j.burns.2020.03.013.

[42] Ma S., Yuan Z., Peng Y., Chen J., Li H., Luo Q. Experience and suggestion of medical practices for burns during the outbreak of COVID-19. Burns. 2020;46(June (4)):749-755. doi: 10.1016/j.burns.2020.03.014.

[43] Corman V.M., Landt O., Kaiser M., Molenkamp R., Meijer A., Chu D.K.W. Detection of 2019 novel coronavirus (2019-nCoV) by real-time RT-PCR. Euro Surveill. 2020 doi: 10.2807/1560-7917.ES.2020.25.3.2000045.

[44] Lauer S.A., Grantz K.H., Bi Q., Jones F.K., Zheng Q., Meredith H. The incubation period of coronavirus disease 2019 (COVID-19) from publicly reported confirmed cases: estimation and application. Ann Intern Med. 2020;(March):1-7. doi: 10.7326/M20-0504